THE ALZHEIMER'S DISEASE CAREGIVER'S HANDBOOK

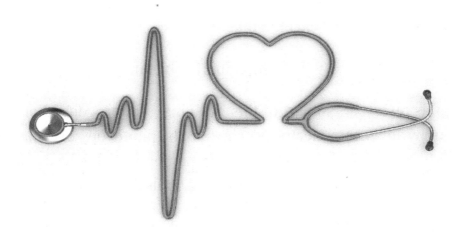

WHAT TO REMEMBER WHEN THEY FORGET

Sally Willard Burbank, M.D.
& Sue Pace Bell

Authors: Dr. Sally Willard Burbank and Sue Pace Bell
Original watercolor artwork: Renee Muha Designs
        Email: **reneemuha@comcast.net**
Cover Artwork: Renee Muha Designs
Cover Designer: Keri Knutson of Alchemy Designs
Vector illustrations and cartoons: Shutterstock and Cartoonstock.com

TABLE OF CONTENTS

PART I

ALZHEIMER'S: THE BASICS

PART II

CARING FOR ALZHEIMER'S PATIENTS

PART III

TAKING CARE OF YOURSELF:

PART IV

HOPE FOR THE FUTURE

PART V

STORIES FROM *Patients I Will Never Forget*

ABOUT THE AUTHORS

Dr. Sally Willard Burbank

Sally Willard Burbank spent her early childhood on a dairy farm in Derby, Vermont, and graduated from Montpelier High School. After graduating summa cum laude from Texas Christian University, she attended medical school at the University of Vermont. Because her husband is a musician, they moved to Nashville in 1986. She completed her internal medicine residency through the University of Tennessee.

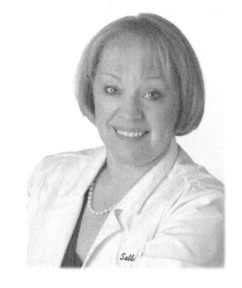

Dr. Burbank and her husband, Nathan, are the proud parents of Steven and Eliza. Sally loves to garden, bicycle, cook, read, and write.

She has six stories published in *Chicken Soup for the Soul*, as well as a book of humorous and touching stories from her experiences as a doctor titled *Patients I Will Never Forget*, which is available from Amazon in paperback and e-book. Three of the stories that relate to Alzheimer's patients are included at the end of this book to provide a little comic relief. She recently completed a romantic comedy called, "Can You Lose the Unibrow?"

Dr. Burbank has practiced internal medicine for thirty years and has diagnosed, doctored, and counseled dozens of Alzheimer's patients and their stressed-out caregivers. In addition, Dr. Burbank's father suffered from mild dementia in the last several years of his life.

Sue Pace Bell

Sue Pace Bell grew up in Waverly, Tennessee, before marrying her high school sweetheart, Ray Bell. Ray coached, taught, and was principal of Waverly Junior High School until he took a job as an agent with State Farm Insurance, where Sue worked as his secretary. They birthed three daughters, and in 1979, Ray became mayor of Waverly.

The Bell's older daughters, Cindy and Renee, married and provided Sue with three wonderful grandchildren: Katie, Jack and Ben.

Sue and Renee opened a jewelry and gift store in Waverly called the Carrollton House, while Ray ran the insurance agency and spent his free time on the golf course.

Two tragedies marred their otherwise ideal life. In 1983, a car accident killed their beautiful 14-year-old daughter, Laura Michelle, and in 2006, Ray received a diagnosis of Alzheimer's disease while still in the prime of life.

Sue quit work to care for him, though she felt unprepared for the daunting responsibility. With experience, she grew comfortable in the role and cared for him until his death on August 20, 2013.

Sue now works a couple of days a week in the gift store and loves spending time with her siblings, children, and grandchildren.

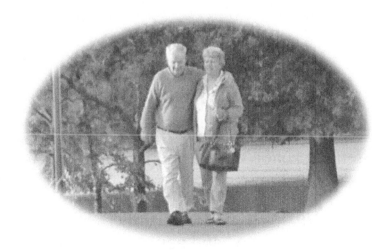

DEDICATION

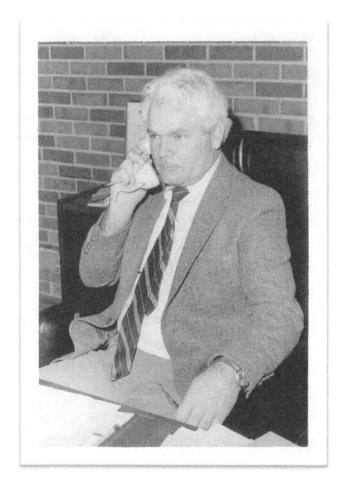

Harold Ray Bell
May 14, 1937 – August 20, 2013
Man of God.
Loving husband and father.
Stellar teacher, coach, and insurance agent.
Golf aficionado and caring friend.
Mayor of Waverly, Tennessee.
Deeply loved and never forgotten.

—

TO OUR READERS:

This book discusses the caregiving of individuals with Alzheimer's disease. A common abbreviation for Alzheimer's disease is AD, and we use this abbreviation throughout the book.

While we focus predominantly on AD, the principles outlined are appropriate for all types of dementia.

We did not write this book with the expectation that caregivers would sit down and read it cover-to-cover like a John Grisham thriller. Rather, we designed it as a guidebook, broken down into topic-specific chapters so a caregiver can flip directly to the subject of greatest relevance on any given day. Because caregivers might read only a few pages at a time—or pull the book out weeks later when the need arrives—information may be repeated when it applies to overlapping areas.

To avoid reading "he or she" repeatedly—which gets tiresome—we have elected to use just one pronoun at a time. The info is applicable to either sex.

The names of patients and caregivers used in this book have been changed to protect patient confidentiality and to comply with all federal HIPAA laws.

Lastly, the advice we offer will not work for every patient, nor is it meant to usurp the advice of your loved one's physician. We offer our best guiding principles, but if they don't work for you or your loved one, don't force it. The success of our advice may also depend on the patient's stage of dementia. Thus, if it doesn't work early on, try it again at a more advanced stage.

Part I provides didactic information about Alzheimer's disease, but if you are only interested in our practical caregiving advice, skip straight to Part II.

In short, glean and apply what is helpful and disregard the rest.

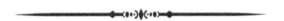

FOREWORD

Throughout your career, you prepare for retirement. You look forward to the day you can relax with the grandchildren, read mysteries, travel to Scotland, plant a garden, or sip tea on the front porch. You scrimp and save for decades so you will have no financial worries in your old age.

Instead, you get flung into the world of progressive dementia. This was not your retirement dream, but it is the hand you were dealt. What now? All your plans—ruined.

An article written years ago by Emily Perl Kingsley described what it felt like when she discovered her child was disabled. It mirrors what it is like to discover your loved one has Alzheimer's. The following story is Emily's analogy:

———◆━◖••◗◆◖••◗━◆———

WELCOME TO HOLLAND

Emily Perl Kingsley

I am often asked to describe the experience of raising a child with a disability—to try to help people who have not shared that unique experience to understand it, to imagine how it would feel. It's like this...

When you're going to have a baby, it's like planning a fabulous vacation trip—to Italy. You buy a bunch of guidebooks and make your wonderful plans. The Coliseum. The Michelangelo David. The gondolas in Venice. You may learn some handy phrases in Italian. It's all very exciting.

After months of eager anticipation, the day finally arrives. You pack your bags and off you go. Several hours later, the plane lands. The flight attendant comes in and says, "Welcome to Holland."

"Holland?!?" you say, "What do you mean Holland?? I signed up for Italy! I'm supposed to be in Italy. All my life I've dreamed of going to Italy."

But there's been a change in the flight plan. They've landed in Holland and there you must stay.

The important thing is that they haven't taken you to a horrible, disgusting, filthy place, full of pestilence, famine and disease. It's just a different place.

So, you must go out and buy new guide books. And you must learn a whole new language. And you will meet a whole new group of people you would never have met.

It's just a *different* place. It's slower-paced than Italy, less flashy than Italy. But after you've been there for a while, you catch your breath, you look around, and you begin to notice that Holland has windmills....and Holland has tulips. Holland even has Rembrandts.

But everyone you know is busy coming and going from Italy, and they're all bragging about what a wonderful time they had there. And for the rest of your life, you will say, "Yes, that's where I was supposed to go. That's what I had planned."

And the pain of that will never, ever, ever, ever go away … because the loss of that dream is a very, very significant loss.

But … if you spend your life mourning the fact that you didn't get to Italy, you may never be free to enjoy the very special, the very lovely things … about Holland.

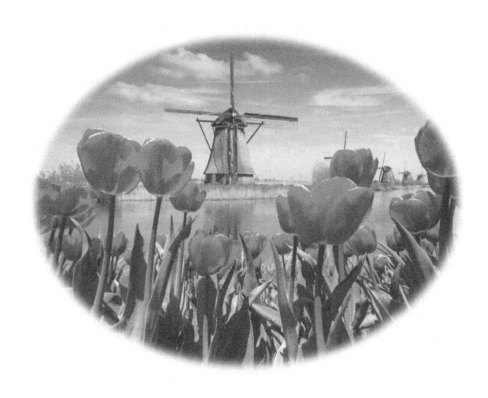

MY STORY

Sue Pace Bell

This book shares the journey I went on with my husband, Ray, who was the love of my life. We were married for fifty-three years, and my journey is similar to that of others who find out their loved one has Alzheimer's.

Two years after my husband retired, he was diagnosed with Alzheimer's, and for the last nine years of his life, I was his caregiver.

I would like to tell you it was easy, but it was full of challenges and, at times, heartache. Because dementia was uncharted territory for me, I felt ill-equipped and scared. Did I have the courage, strength, and knowledge to endure what lay ahead?

My husband and I had planned for our retirement for decades. We had worked hard and diligently saved money. We eagerly anticipated our "golden years" as a blissful time of traveling to Europe, exploring new golf courses, and planning fun-filled adventures with our grandchildren. Because of Alzheimer's, however, our journey was not what we had planned. No dining in five-star restaurants, no trips to Paris or Prague. No strolling through the Disney castle with our grandchildren, as I couldn't risk losing Ray into a huge crowd if I turned my back for two seconds.

Our journey was sometimes frightening, sometimes difficult, and often confusing. Many times, I wasn't sure how to handle what was thrust upon me. Where do I get help? Who could tell me how to handle this particular problem? The day-to-day responsibility, worry, and second-guessing was mentally and physically exhausting.

If you are faced with a similar journey, it will be the most challenging journey you ever take, even though you won't be traveling anywhere. I can liken your journey to sailing on a ship.

Some days, when the winds are blustery, the waves will be stormy and rough. Other days, when the water is calm, and the sun is shining, you will have smooth sailing and an enjoyable day. For some caregiveres, the journey will be short with the shoreline clearly in sight. Others will feel as though they are sailing for months on end with no lighthouse on the horizon to guide them.

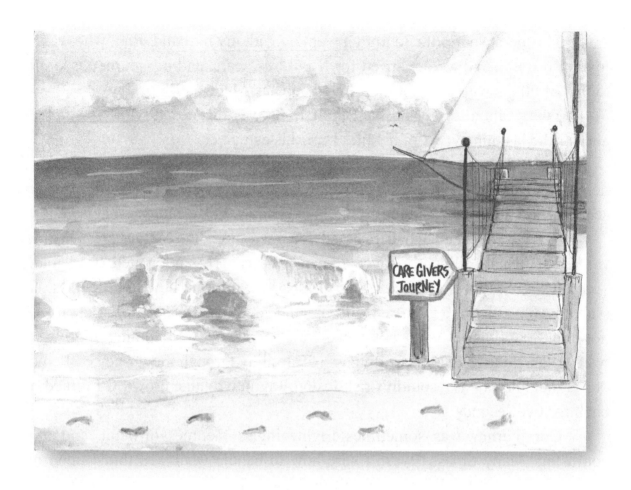

If you are like me, you like to prepare for trips. When I travel to someplace new, I purchase travel guides and road maps. I talk to people who have been there. I pack appropriate clothing and schedule my time to best utilize my vacation days. My journey with Alzheimer's disease provided no such guidebooks, and I often felt like I was being jostled by choppy waves with no coastline in sight and no compass to guide me.

This book—a travel guide of sorts—is written to help you prepare for and navigate through the unpredictable waters of dementia. So many times, I wished I'd had a blueprint to tell me what to expect next and how to handle a challenging situation.

Instead, I muddled through, as best I could, learning mostly by trial and error. Thus, I offer this book as my footprint to help you successfully provide care for your loved one with Alzheimer's or some other type of dementia. I am sharing everything I learned the hard way.

Unfortunately, once you set sail on this journey, there is no turning back, and while I have included signposts of what to expect along the way, no two journeys will be alike.

It is my hope, however, that this book will smooth your sailing and make your journey less turbulent. Greet each day knowing others have taken this trip before you and survived. You can too!

REFLECTIONS
Dr. Sally Burbank

In the quarter of a century I have practiced internal medicine, I have diagnosed and treated my share of patients with dementia. During these years, I have helped dozens of families navigate the perilous waters of Alzheimer's disease. Some caregivers never seem to grasp that their loved one is physically unable to remember what they are told. The caregiver acts perpetually frustrated and "put out" with the patient. Some accuse the patient of purposely forgetting or acting irresponsibly.

On rare occasions, I have witnessed the ugly side and have had to intervene when the patient's health was in jeopardy due to neglect or abuse, both physical and mental. I've seen patients left lying in nursing home beds for years with no family or visitors. They are drugged up and kept alive on tube feeding, long past the point where they can talk or recognize family. They develop bedsores and require urine catheters. Many have nightmares that leave them terrified and hollering in the night because they can't separate dreams from reality.

Thankfully, I have also had the joy of working with dozens of caregivers, such as Sue Bell and my mother, who handled their loved one's dementia with patience, common sense, and a positive attitude.

I have asked myself, "What did Sue Bell and my mother do differently than the caregivers who either act like martyrs or become overwhelmed with the daunting responsibility? How were Sue and my mother able to roll with the punches and still maintain an upbeat attitude and calm demeanor?

In the nine years that Sue took care of her husband, Ray, I remember telling myself that I needed to interview her and glean as much as I could about caring for a loved one with Alzheimer's disease. How did she do it, day in and day out, without losing her joy, let alone her sanity? Sue's ability to handle situations with aplomb was truly inspiring. She somehow found a way to not let caregiving swallow her up whole. Instead, she intentionally carved out time for herself, enlisted the help of family and friends, and found ways to "have a life," even though her days of caregiving were long and demanding.

After her husband passed, I approached Sue about writing a book together—a practical guide for those whose loved ones have dementia.

In this book, we share not only the wisdom Sue learned the hard way, but also the collective knowledge of nurses at assisted living facilities, memory care centers, and nursing homes. We interviewed successful caregivers and compiled their best advice to create this caregiver's guide.

I have also included my best advice from years of practicing internal medicine, as well as the tidbits I have gleaned from reading dozens of books about caregiving Alzheimer's patients. I hope you find it helpful.

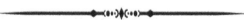

To provide a better understanding of Alzheimer's disease, Part I includes general information about the disease itself. Part II delves into caregiving, and Part III discusses how to take care of yourself in the midst of a demanding role. Part IV provides a brief summary of ongoing research to cure this dreaded disease. I end with three humorous stories about Alzheimer's patients taken from my book, *Patients I Will Never Forget.*

Obviously, there is no "one-size-fits-all" approach to dementia, but we hope the tips and suggestions we provide will make your journey through the murky waters of Alzheimer's less stressful.

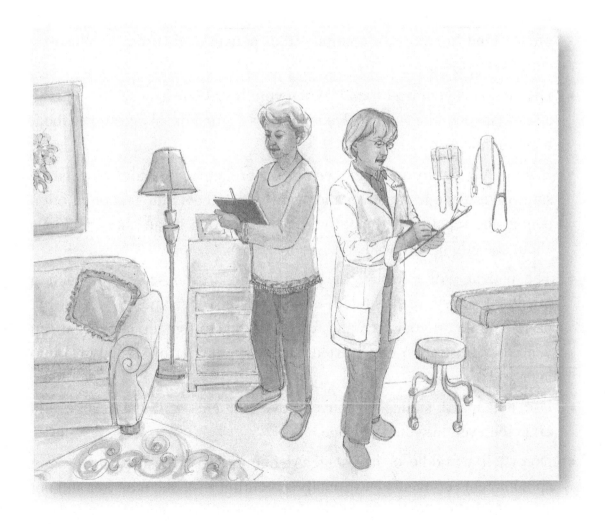

CAREGIVER PEARLS

Dr. Sally Burbank

- Don't try to orient the patient back to reality—it only agitates her. Instead, put yourself in her world and her mind. For example, avoid statements like, "No, Mom, your sister died ten years ago," or, "You *are* home—*this* is your home!" Far better to get Mom talking about the sister she remembers—and still thinks is alive—or the childhood home she loved.

- Focus on the activities the patient still *can* do, and do those activities often. Find a way to continue the patient's favorite hobbies by simplifying them.

- Distraction is your best friend. When your loved one is upset, try singing a familiar song like "Old McDonald Had a Farm," or ask questions about her childhood.

- If your AD family member becomes a broken record and repeats the same phrase or question over and over, try to uncover the fear or emotion behind the repetition. Repetitive questions often mean she is anxious about something and needs reassurance.

- The patient will mirror your emotions and responses. Avoid acting impatient, angry, or frustrated, or she may also become upset. Instead, paste a smile on your face and force yourself to remain calm. You can vent your frustration to a trusted friend or member of a support group later.

- Use touch and smiles to convey love. Patients still crave love and affection even into the last stage.

- Don't tell a middle or late-stage Alzheimer's patient about upcoming appointments or events—especially at bedtime—or she may fret and not sleep. Alzheimer's disease skews her sense of time, and she may dress for church at 3 a.m. or insist an upcoming birthday party you casually mentioned yesterday will occur today—for three weeks straight!

- Find humor whenever and wherever you can.

- Invest in adult pull-ups when incontinence becomes a problem. Replace all underwear in the drawer with disposable ones. Use elastic waistband pants in a size larger than normal to make removal easier. In early Alzheimer's, timed voiding every two to three hours minimizes accidents. Use a "double diaper" technique when out in public.

- Place a fully charged cellphone with a "Find My Phone" app in the patient's pocket every morning. Obtain a Safe Return bracelet from the Alzheimer's Association.

- Find pleasure living in the moment. Enjoy hummingbirds at the birdfeeder, the scent of a beautiful rose, the soft fur of a friendly kitty, the giggle of a baby, or the taste of a fresh peach. Until the last stage, patients enjoy these sensory pleasures and can still find joy in life. As a caregiver, make a point of appreciating the simple things each day.

- Help your loved one communicate by filling in the missing word she can't remember or by asking her to describe what she is trying to say. The goal is to keep her communicating as long as possible. Don't force her to try to come up with the forgotten word if she can't remember it, or she may get frustrated and quit trying or forget the rest of her story.

- Don't ask the patient if she *wants* to go to the Senior Citizen's Center for lunch, or to daycare or church: she may resist social events because they frighten her. Even if she went last week and had a great time, she won't *remember* she had a great time and may therefore resist. Don't give advance warning by asking, or she may fret and argue until you cave in and decide not to go. Instead, merely tell her you are going for a drive. Leave a little early and drive around town looking at houses and points of interest. Then, "spontaneously" stop at the church or Senior Citizen's

Center. By not providing advanced warning, she doesn't have time to argue or worry.

- If the patient refuses to get out of the car, don't argue. Instead, calmly pick up her legs and swing them around to the outside of the car. Stay calm and pleasant and start singing her favorite childhood song to distract her. Caregivers waste too much time trying to talk patients into things. Just do it!

- Never rely on the patient's memory to remember what you tell her. Instead, leave large notes with pictures in plain sight such as, "In the garden" or, "In the bathtub," or "Gone to the store. Back by 11:00." Draw a clock with the hands pointing to 11:00.

- Break complex tasks—such as taking a bath—into simple, one-step instructions. If she resists, don't push it. Instead, try again a few minutes later.

- Offer two choices whenever possible, knowing she will likely pick the second option. This allows your patient to have some sense of control.

- Don't let the patient nod off all day in her chair or she won't sleep well at night. To encourage sleeping at night, keep the patient physically and mentally active during the day, and take her outside in the bright light every morning, weather permitting. Maintain consistent times for getting up and going to bed.

- Carry business cards that say, "She has dementia. Thanks for understanding." These can be discretely handed out if she acts up in public. Most people will nod and smile once they understand the reason for the strange behavior.

- Create a schedule that includes one hour of "me" time for the caregiver. You need something to look forward to every day.

- Educate family and friends not to argue with or to correct the patient. Ask them to remind the patient who they are and their connection to the patient. Example: "Hi, George. It's Carol Bates. We used to sing in the church choir together."

- Find trusted and reliable people to help you. AD is a marathon not a sprint, so you cannot do it by yourself without straining your own health. You will have to *ask* for help, as people will not volunteer on their own. Be specific with your need, such as, "I need someone to sit with George on Saturday from 10-11 so I can get a haircut." Give plenty of notice so helpers can mark it in their calendars. Reward or pay volunteers for their time, or at least insist on covering the cost of their gas.

- Take caregiving one day at a time. If you look too far in the future, it feels overwhelming. Jesus said, "One day's worry is enough for one day." Pray for the strength and wisdom to make it through this one day.

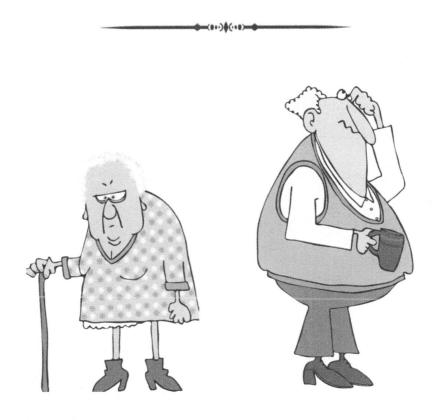

PART I

ALZHEIMER'S: THE BASICS

CHAPTER 1

—●··◦)◦(··◦—

UNDERSTANDING ALZHEIMER'S

Dr. Sally Burbank

What is Alzheimer's disease?

Alzheimer's is a brain disease that progressively destroys memory and judgment. In its severest stage, patients are unable to independently perform the simplest tasks of daily living, such as bathing, eating, and dressing. They may not recognize or remember their own spouse and children yet may retain memories from their childhood.

The term "Alzheimer's disease" dates back to 1906, when a German physician, Dr. Alois Alzheimer, presented the case of a demented 51-year-old whose brain autopsy revealed abnormal clumps (called amyloid plaques) and tangled bundles of nerve fibers (called neurofibrillary tangles). These two anatomical abnormalities, along with a loss of connections between nerve cells, are considered proof positive that a patient has Alzheimer's and not one of the alternative causes of dementia.

How prevalent is the disease?

Estimates vary as to how many people have Alzheimer's. Most put the total at 5.5 million in the United States. As the baby boom generation ages, however, this number is projected to skyrocket. Why? Because the likelihood of developing the disease increases exponentially after the age of sixty-five. The average life span after diagnosis is around seven years, though this varies greatly.

Alzheimer's disease is the most common cause of dementia in people aged sixty-five and older, and it is the fifth leading cause of death in senior adults. More people die of Alzheimer's each year in the United States than of breast cancer and prostate cancer combined. In fact, *one in nine people over the age of sixty-five will*

---

develop Alzheimer's, and thus, over half of us will, at some point in our lives, help care for a parent, spouse, sibling, or in-law with Alzheimer's. Since Medicare does not cover assisted living facilities or extended nursing home stays, *85 percent of the care provided to patients with AD is provided by family.* The hours spent by family members caring for loved ones with AD is financially uncompensated. Thus, it is critical for families to be educated about Alzheimer's and to be equipped to competently care for patients at each stage of the disease.

How does aging affect the incidence of Alzheimer's?

Alzheimer's disease is not a normal part of aging, as only half of those who live to the age of 100 develop the disease. However, the greatest risk factor for developing Alzheimer's is increasing age. Since the average lifespan of Americans has increased to over eighty, the risk of AD has increased significantly, as the chart below shows:

Age	Prevalence of AD
Younger than 65	3%
65-70	4%
71-79	5%
80-84	13.5%
85-89	31%
90-94	40%
Older than 95	53%

How does the brain work? What goes wrong in AD?

Your brain weighs only three pounds, but it is the control center for the entire body. A healthy brain has 100 billion active nerve cells and is nourished through a vast network of blood vessels.

The brain receives information from the rest of the body and then makes decisions based on the information it receives. This information is gathered through our five senses—vision, hearing, smell, taste, and touch—then transmitted through nerve cells up the spinal cord to the brain.

There are three major parts to the brain. The brain stem connects the brain to the spinal cord and controls automatic responses in the body like breathing. The cerebrum allows a person to think, feel, and remember. The cerebellum controls balance. See the diagram below:

Major Parts of the Brain

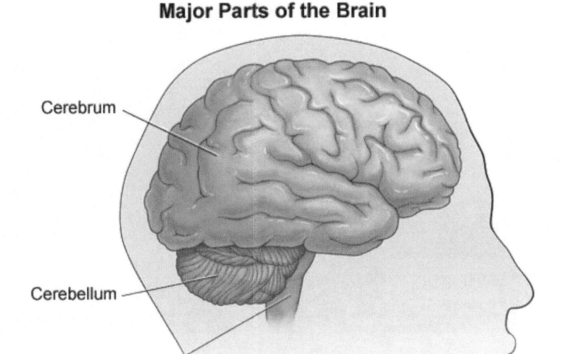

As can be seen in the following diagram, different parts of the cerebrum are responsible for different functions, such as vision, hearing, moving, speech, and touch.

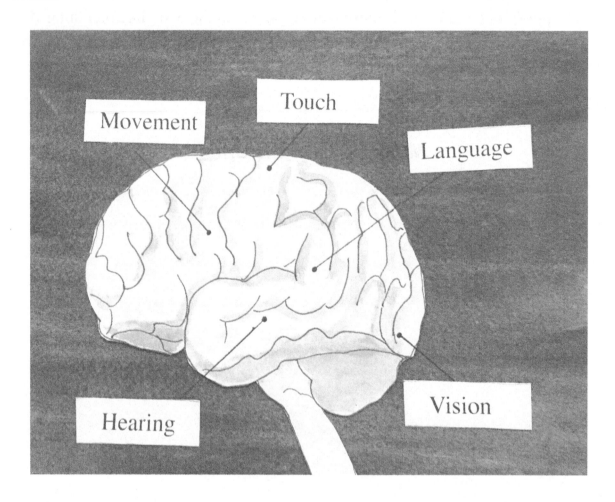

AD causes the cerebrum to shrink due to progressive death of nerve cells. The shrinkage is especially severe in the hippocampus, a small, seahorse-shaped area of the cortex located in the temporal lobe. This small structure is critical in forming new memories. Thus, when the hippocampus shrinks, short-term memory becomes seriously impaired. See the following diagram:

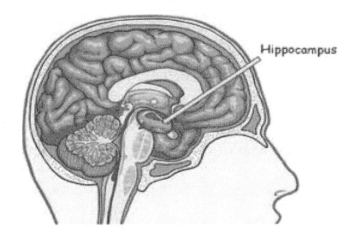

Below is a cross-section of a healthy brain versus one shrunken from advanced Alzheimer's disease.

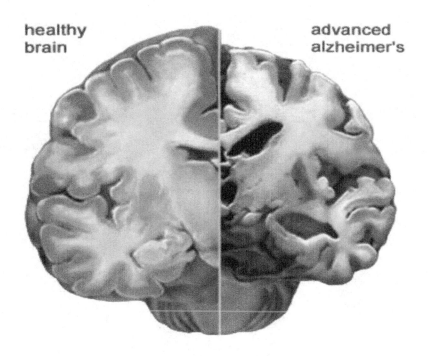

In AD, abnormal beta-amyloid proteins called amyloid plaques form sticky clumps between nerve cells in the brain and interfere with the communication between cells. By interfering with the nerve cell's ability to send and receive messages, the brain cell gradually dies. As more and more brain cells die, the brain shrinks.

In addition to damage *between* cells caused by *amyloid plaques*, damage also occurs *within* individual nerve cells due to the accumulation of an abnormal protein that interferes with the smooth flow of nutrition within the cell. These *neurofibrillary tangles*, made up of tau protein, ultimately lead to the death of the nerve cell.

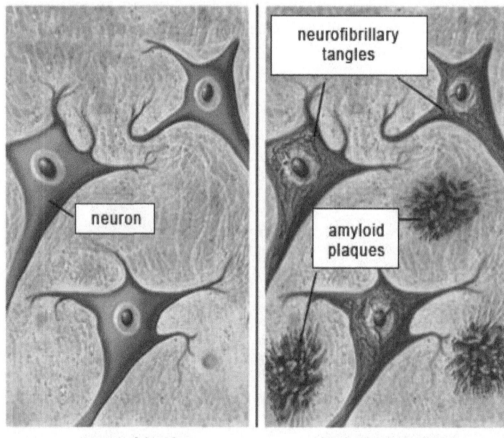

normal brain   Alzheimer's brain

Is Alzheimer's always a downward trajectory?

Unfortunately, yes. While there are effective treatments for many other diseases, Alzheimer's is particularly heartbreaking because there is no cure, and even the best medications merely slow its downward progression.

If a person has a broken leg and hobbles around on crutches, you can see his disability and extend patience when he delays you getting off the elevator. When someone has AD, however, it is not necessarily obvious, so people often don't understand or make allowances for unusual behavior. Likewise, you wouldn't expect a toddler, whose brain isn't fully matured, to understand advanced calculus equations because you know abstract math is outside his age-appropriate abilities. Even though we cannot always *see* the disability of an AD patient, we must learn to extend the same patience and understanding that we offer to those with more obvious limitations.

While a broken bone heals, and a child's brain matures, the opposite is true for those with Alzheimer's—their condition gradually spirals further and further down. With each passing year they lose more and more of their mental and physical abilities. They may seem to plateau for a while, but it is always a downward trajectory, and once a cognitive or physical skill is lost, it will not be regained.

If the brain is compared to a computer, the AD patient's brain can no longer transmit information properly. Certain links become permanently damaged, and more parts of the brain become inoperable. It is as though AD inserts a virus into the computer of the brain and gradually makes the brain unable to function. Remind yourself that your loved one doesn't mean to be annoying; he is doing the best he can with a malfunctioning brain.

Shrunken Language and
Memory Centers in an Alzheimer's Brain

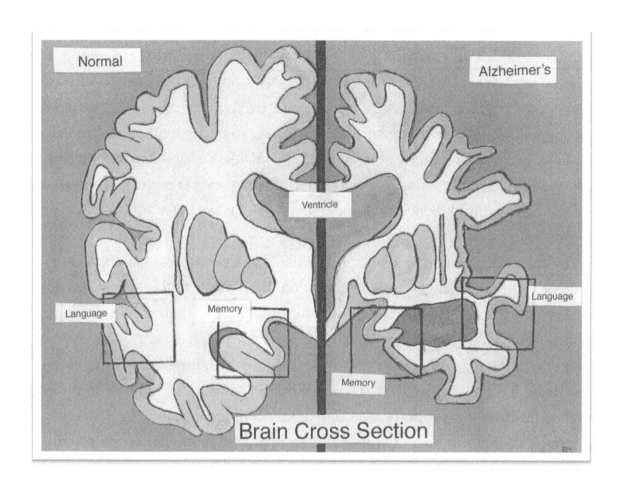

CHAPTER 2

❖

WHAT CAUSES ALZHEIMER'S?

Dr. Sally Burbank

The Genetics of Alzheimer's

Five percent of Alzheimer's sufferers are diagnosed before age sixty. The vast majority of these early-onset patients have inherited a genetic mutation on chromosome 1, 14, or 21, which accounts for their early onset of disease. Early-onset AD can begin as early as age thirty and will advance toward end-stage disease more quickly than late-onset Alzheimer's. These unfortunate individuals usually have other family members with early-onset Alzheimer's.

Half of those with late-onset Alzheimer's disease—meaning those over age sixty-five when diagnosed—have inherited what is called a gene "allele" on chromosome 19 called APO lipoprotein E4. Research suggests having one or two copies of the APO E4 gene increases your risk of Alzheimer's. Let me explain:

Everyone inherits two copies of an APO E gene allele—one from their mother and one from their father. The APO E gene provides a blueprint to a protein that carries cholesterol in the blood. This APO E gene comes in three different allele forms: APO E2, APO E3, and APO E4.

Those fortunate enough to carry two copies of APO E2 (<1 percent of the population) are protected completely from developing AD. Those with one copy of E2 have a 40 percent *reduced* rate of Alzheimer's. APO E3, the gene form that 61 percent of us carry, is neutral. That is, it neither raises nor lowers your risk.

APO E4, however, is a bad actor. If you inherit one copy of this gene from one of your parents, your risk for AD is *tripled*. If you inherit the APO E4 gene from b*oth* parents, your risk increases to a whopping *ten times normal*. It doesn't mean you are doomed to get AD, but your risk is markedly increased compared to someone with E2 or E3 alleles.

In fact, some researchers estimate that 55 percent of those with late-onset Alzheimer's disease have at least one copy of the APO E4 gene. An estimated 25 percent of Americans carry at least one copy of the APO E4 gene, but thankfully, only 2 percent carry two copies of the dreaded gene.

Distribution of E2, E3, and E4 Alleles and the Risk for AD

% with Allele	Inheritance of APO E	Risk for AD
<1%	E2/E2	0 % Risk
11%	E2/E3	Risk decreased by 40%
61%	E3/E3	Average Risk
2%	E2/E4	Average Risk
23%	E3/E4	Risk is tripled
2%	E4/E4	Risk is increased 10-times

Adding to the confusion, not everyone who carries two APO E4 alleles will develop Alzheimer's—they are just at ten-times greater risk.

Furthermore, if one identical twin develops AD, the risk of the other twin developing it is only 45%, and if both identical twins develop AD, one twin may develop the disease a full decade later than the first twin, even though they carry identical genes. Thus, environmental factors play an equally important role.

Research has shown, for example, that those with APO-E4 alleles raise their already heightened risk of AD even more if they smoke, have an elevated LDL cholesterol, or an elevated blood pressure in midlife. Thus, controlling blood pressure, following a Mediterranean diet (see below), quitting smoking, and staying trim and in shape, are critical for those who inherit APO E4 genes.

What environmental factors increase risk of Alzheimer's?

Smoking, high blood pressure, high LDL cholesterol, midlife obesity, a junk food diet rich in trans fats, isolation or lack of daily social interactions, sedentary lifestyle, and lower educational achievement—all increase the risk for AD.

Having a mentally challenging job that includes plenty of interaction with other people lowers the risk, as does aerobic exercise and regular participation in at least three social clubs or groups. Thus, many risk factors for AD are modifiable.

What we eat is critically important. One large, prospective study showed that those who adhered strictly to a Mediterranean diet—a diet rich in salmon, tuna, olive oil, colorful vegetables, fruits, nuts, legumes, whole grains, red grapes, and one or two glasses of red wine daily—throughout their adulthood had a 40 percent decreased risk of Alzheimer's compared to those who ate diets devoid of the healthy foods listed above.

Some scientists have focused on DHA (docosahexaenoic acid), an omega-3 fatty acid found in salmon and other fatty fish. Studies performed on mice genetically predisposed to AD revealed that diets rich in DHA reduced beta-amyloid plaques in the brains of these mice. Although a clinical trial of DHA supplements showed no impact on humans with mild to moderate Alzheimer's disease, it is likely that the DHA supplements were started too late in the disease process to be effective. Studies are ongoing to see if fish oil supplements started much sooner—long before cognitive symptoms appear—might be helpful. Until this is proven, to lower your risk of Alzheimer's, follow the Mediterranean diet as

—

early in life as possible, because once the disease has manifested itself, it may be too late for diet changes or fish oil supplements to make much of a difference.

What about the Mediterranean Diet?

The Mediterranean diet is a diet inspired by the eating habits of Greece, Southern Italy, and Spain. It is widely recognized as promoting health and well-being. The main aspects of the diet include proportionally high consumption of olive oil, fish, legumes, unrefined cereals, colorful fruits, and vegetables, nuts, moderate consumption of dairy products (mostly as cheese and yogurt), moderate red wine consumption, and *low* consumption of red meats and processed foods (which are high in trans fats). Some researchers believe olive oil may be the main health-promoting component of the diet. There is preliminary evidence showing regular consumption of olive oil may lower the risk of cancer, cardiovascular disease, brain degeneration (including AD), and several other chronic diseases.

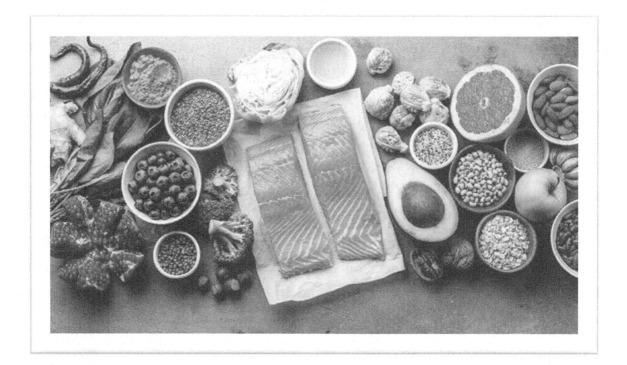

What about vitamins and supplements?

One area of research is focusing on antioxidants, which are natural substances that fight damage caused by free radicals. As we age, free radicals build up in our nerve cells causing damage that might contribute to AD. Several epidemiological and laboratory studies suggest that antioxidants from food or dietary supplements may help prevent this oxidative damage, and thus, lower the risk of Alzheimer's. Most studies, however, have shown no benefit from vitamins. Vitamins C, B, ginkgo biloba, and Co-Q-10 have all been thoroughly tested in clinical trials and proven useless in preventing or slowing the progression of AD.

Resveratrol, a compound found in red grapes and wine, may help protect the brain. Observational studies have shown that moderate consumption of red wine is associated with a lower incidence of Alzheimer's disease, and animal studies have shown that resveratrol can reduce beta-amyloid deposits in the brain. Resveratrol appears to affect age-related diseases, including Alzheimer's. An NIH-supported clinical trial is currently underway to test the effects of resveratrol in people with Alzheimer's disease, but the results aren't back yet. For now, eating red grapes or drinking grape juice or red wine in controlled quantities (no more than ten 6-oz glasses of wine per week in women and fourteen glasses per week in men) couldn't hurt. Obviously, those who struggle with alcoholism shouldn't drink at all. Twelve ounces of wine per day is the maximum for men, ten ounces for women.

Data from one randomized, controlled study showed taking Vitamin E 1000 IU twice a day may be beneficial for those with mild to moderate dementia. A 2014 study by Dysken, Dano, and Asthana (JAMA 2014; 311 (11): 1161) showed that those who received Vitamin E 1,000 IU twice a day had a slower decline in functional status (3.15 points less decline than those on a placebo on a 78-point scale over four years). Vitamin E delayed functional decline by 6.2 months, and patients on Vitamin E required less caregiver time compared to the placebo group. All the participants in this study were veterans who were also receiving a cholinesterase inhibitor Alzheimer's medication (such as Aricept) to treat their disease. Vitamin E has not yet been shown to *prevent* AD.

What about exercise?

Aerobic exercise and increased physical activity are protective to the brain. In a study of 716 senior citizens with an average age of eighty-two, the ten percent least physically active seniors were 2.3 times more likely to develop Alzheimer's disease compared to the 10 percent most active seniors. Brain-helping activity included housework, yard work, walking to the mailbox, and daily walks. Just don't sit in a chair all day watching television or playing computer games. Be as physically active as you are able.

How does exercise help? Researchers have shown that aerobic exercise stimulates the brain's ability to maintain old network connections and to form *new* ones that are vital to healthy cognition. In a year-long study, sixty-five older people exercised daily doing either an aerobic exercise program of walking forty minutes a day or a non-aerobic program of stretching and toning exercises. At the end of the trial, the walking group showed improved connectivity in the part of the brain engaged in daydreaming, envisioning the future, and recalling the past. The walking group also improved on executive function (the ability to plan and organize tasks such as cooking a meal). In short, try to get a total of forty minutes a day of aerobic activity, such as walking, swimming, bicycling on a stationary exercise bike, or taking classes at the YMCA.

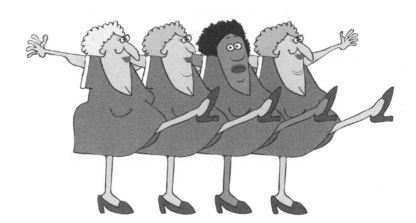

Will doing crossword puzzles prevent dementia?

Brain-challenging activities and learning new skills can delay the progression of Alzheimer's by as much as four to five years. Take up a new hobby like playing the guitar or learning how to play Bridge. Learn to crochet. Play Scrabble or Words with Friends. Solve Sudokus or challenging crossword puzzles. Do jigsaw puzzles. Challenge your brain with NEW activities, as these are more likely to stimulate the brain than always resorting to your familiar hobbies.

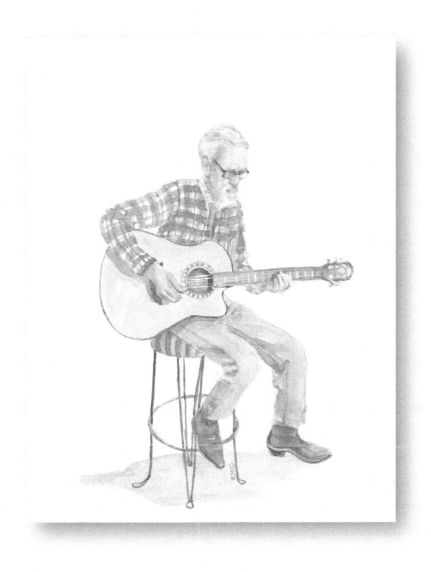

For fun, try using your non-dominant hand to move your computer mouse or to eat meals. Join a canasta or bridge club. Sign up for ballroom dancing and practice intricate dance steps. Visit museums and art galleries. Watch PBS or the History Channel and try to recount to your friends what you learn.

Take up a foreign language. Studies show bilingual individuals have lower rates of dementia, and one of the best stimulations to the brain is to learn a new language as an adult. Buy a Rosetta Stone CD or download a language-learning app like Duolingo. If possible, practice speaking the language with someone native to that tongue. Try to memorize new words and phrases until you become fluent.

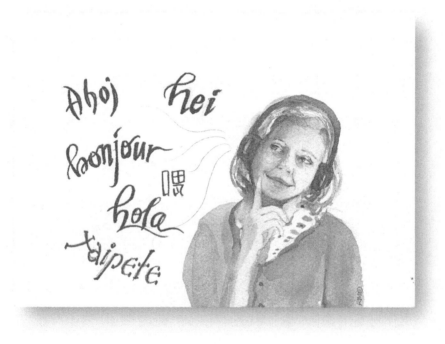

Purchase a yearly membership to Lumosity.com and commit to brain-stimulating games each day. Even mundane activities, like going to the grocery store, can provide a brain challenge. Try to memorize five items on your grocery list and see if you can remember them by the time you get to the store. Gradually increase the number of grocery items you commit to memory until you can retain six or seven items.

What else can I do to prevent Alzheimer's?

Stay socially active. After you retire, don't sit home watching TV and playing computer games all day. Keep active in church, clubs, charities, or travel outings. Join a Bridge club. Play games with your family. Engaging in regular conversation stimulates the brain even more than reading a book. Why? Conversing with others forces us to focus and to think of the word we are trying to say. This stimulates the short-term memory center of the brain.

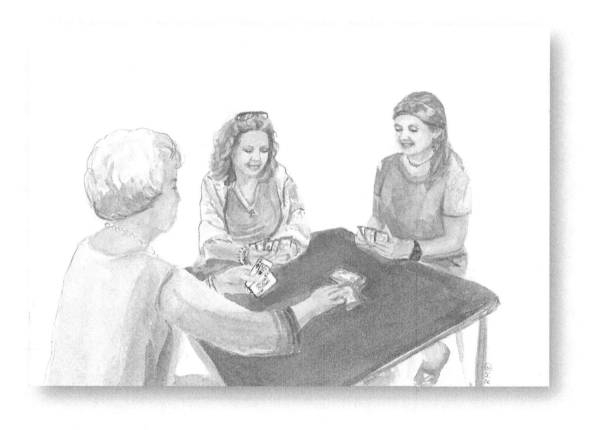

Make sleep a priority. Adequate sleep is vital for forming and processing memories. Chronic sleep deprivation and stress inhibit the normal sequence of memory formation between the hippocampus and cerebral cortex. To aide in falling asleep, maintain consistent bedtimes and get-up times. Try reading before bed instead of sitting in front of bright television or computer screens. Avoid upsetting news programs or arguments at night.

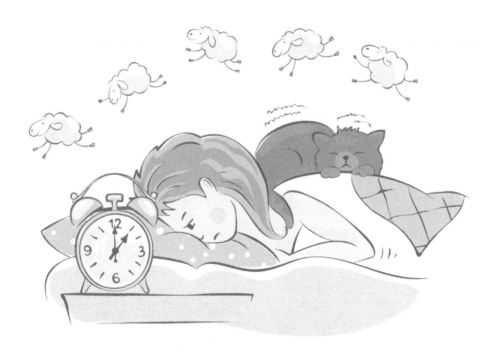

CHAPTER 3

ALZHEIMER'S AND OTHER CAUSES OF DEMENTIA

Dr. Sally Burbank

Are Alzheimer's and dementia interchangeable terms?

No. While Alzheimer's disease is the most *common* cause of dementia (60-70 percent), there are many other conditions that cause dementia.

What are other causes of dementia?

Vascular Dementia: Vascular dementia is the second most common cause of dementia, and it results from impaired blood flow to the brain. This can occur after a large stroke or repeated tiny lacunar strokes. Vascular dementia often progresses in a step-like fashion with a noticeable decline after each mini-stroke followed by a period of stability followed by another decline with the next mini-stroke.

Frontotemporal Dementia (FTD) or Pick's Disease: Pick's disease specifically attacks the frontal and temporal lobes of the brain. It typically starts between ages fifty and sixty. Pick's disease causes drastic personality changes, as well as deterioration of social skills and a lack of empathy and emotions. The patient's ability to speak deteriorates. The undesirable personality changes occur *before* serious memory problems. This differentiates it from AD.

Creutzfeldt-Jakob Disease (CJD): Also known as "mad cow disease," CJD is caused by virus-like particles called prions. Ten percent of cases have a genetic link, but it is usually caused by contaminated meat or infected medical equipment. This disease progresses rapidly and distinguishes itself from Alzheimer's by its rapid progression.

Head Trauma and Repetitive Concussions: Veterans, athletes, and those with severe head trauma are predisposed. The injury can be from one severe head trauma (i.e. car accident or war injury) or from repeated blows to the brain (i.e. football players, boxers, etc.).

Huntington's Chorea: This rare, inherited disease typically presents when the patient is in his forties or fifties. The patient displays bizarre jerking arm movements called chorea. Since the disease is autosomal dominant, the patient must have a mother or father who genetically passed the disease on to them, though the parent could have died before manifesting symptoms of the disease. Genetic testing can positively identify or eliminate Huntington's as a cause of dementia.

Lewy Body Dementia: In Lewy body dementia, deposits of an abnormal brain protein called alpha-synuclein gets deposited inside brain cells. Patients with this disease present with behavioral problems, vivid visual hallucinations, fluctuating alertness, and severe sleep problems, including acting out one's dreams or making severe involuntary movements while asleep.

Normal Pressure Hydrocephalus: NPH is caused by an abnormal increase in cerebral spinal fluid in the brain's cavities, which puts pressure on the brain. In addition to dementia, patients with NPH suffer from incontinence and impaired balance when walking. Frequent falls are common. It is treated with a brain shunt to reduce the amount of spinal fluid in the brain.

Parkinson's disease: Parkinson's is known more for tremor, rigidity, and balance issues, but cognitive decline can also occur late in the disease.

General Anesthesia: Multiple surgeries requiring general anesthesia over the span of two or three years—especially if they are back-to-back—increase the risk of dementia. Coronary artery bypass grafting (CABG) seems to especially trigger cognitive decline in some patients.

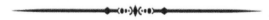

CHAPTER 4

WHAT ARE THE SYMPTOMS OF ALZHEIMER'S?

Dr. Sally Burbank

The symptoms of Alzheimer's change significantly as the disease progresses. Short-term memory loss predominates in the early stages of AD, while complete inability to be self-sufficient predominates in the later stages. Moderate AD falls halfway in between and has a slow, downward trajectory. Here are the major symptoms you should expect with Alzheimer's, and the severity of these symptoms will worsen as the disease progresses:

Memory Loss that Disrupts Daily Life

The best-known symptom of Alzheimer's disease is short-term memory loss. The patient cannot remember what you told her five minutes ago. Other impairments include forgetting appointments or showing up on the wrong day; asking for the same information over and over; having to rely on memory aids (reminder notes, electronic devices, family members) for things she used to just remember; and difficulty reading a book because she can't retain the characters or the plot. As the disease progresses to moderately severe, she will forget the faces and names of close family members and friends. By late stage, she won't even recognize *herself* in the mirror. She will forget her address and phone number. In early AD, she won't know the day of the week; later on, she won't know the month or year.

What's normal? Forgetting the name of someone you should know, but when reminded, you think, "Of course!" Many times, the forgotten name or word will come to you later. Forgetting one of your many computer passwords is normal.

Inability to Plan or Solve Problems

Patients will experience changes in their ability to develop and follow a plan or to perform simple calculations. They may have trouble following a familiar recipe ("Did I already add the salt?") or using the riding lawn mower. They may have difficulty staying focused, and thus take longer to complete tasks. Often, their calculations in the checkbook are wrong, and bounced checks may occur.

What's normal? Making occasional subtraction errors in the checkbook and rare scatterbrained "senior moments," especially when distracted, tired, or stressed.

Difficulty Completing Familiar Tasks

People with Alzheimer's find it hard to complete daily tasks, such as preparing meals, taking medications properly, wearing clean and appropriate clothes, and basic hygiene. Left on their own, in later stages, they may never bathe because they don't remember when they last took a bath or shower. They look disheveled and seem content to wear the same food-stained outfit for days on end. The fly of their pants may be down, and the buttons on their shirt or blouse may be fastened improperly. They may have trouble driving to a familiar location without getting lost—especially at night. They can't retain the rules to a favorite card game.

What's normal? Needing help to navigate the settings on your DVD, cell phone, or computer, or getting lost in a new location or a place you haven't been to in a while.

Confusion with Time, Place, or Person

People with Alzheimer's disease often get lost because they don't recognize previously familiar landmarks. They may not recognize the face of people they should know and often don't remember when they last ate or showered.

What's normal? Getting temporarily confused about the day of the week. You should always recognize and know the names of your spouse, children, and close friends. Not remembering the names of casual acquaintances is normal.

Trouble with Visual Images and Spatial Relationships

In AD, judging distances and determining color or contrast becomes a challenge. Thus, fender benders when driving are common. In late-stage AD, the patient may pass a mirror and think someone else is in the room because he doesn't recognize his own reflection. He may think his wife is his mother because his memory of his wife is from a much younger time period when she wasn't old and gray. Memories of grandchildren get stuck at a young age, and the ability to grasp that grandchildren grow from babies to children to teenagers to adults doesn't register. They may talk proudly about their granddaughter, but not realize that the beautiful college student sitting in front of them *is* that granddaughter.

What's normal? Not recognizing someone you haven't seen in years, especially if they have put on weight, changed their hairstyle, or become bald.

Problems with Words

People with Alzheimer's have trouble following a conversation. They may stop in the middle of their story and have no idea what they were going to say or what point they were trying to make. They ask the same question over and over and don't remember the answer you provided five minutes ago. They may struggle with naming objects and finding the right word in a conversation. They may call things by the wrong name (e.g., calling a watch a "hand clock").

What's normal? Occasionally having trouble coming up with the right word on the spur of the moment in the middle of a conversation. It is also normal to occasionally lose your train of thought and forget what you were going to say. It will usually come to you later.

Misplacing Things and Losing the Ability to Retrace Steps

A person with Alzheimer's disease may put things in unusual places. They may lose things and not be able to retrace their steps to find them. They will often become suspicious and accuse others of stealing the misplaced item. This occurs more frequently as the disease progresses. They may accuse a loved one of stealing their money since they don't remember spending it.

What's normal? Occasionally misplacing things, such as a pair of eyeglasses, the car keys, or the remote control, especially if you were distracted when you set the item down. Once you find it, you will usually remember having put it there.

Poor Judgment

People with Alzheimer's may experience changes in judgment or decision-making. They may give large amounts of money to telemarketers or con artists that claim they are from the IRS or a local bank. Ironically, while they may accuse a loving daughter of stealing their money, they often fall prey to the lies of scammers. They pay less attention to grooming and hygiene. They may leave the house on a cold day with no sweater or coat and drive to the store in their bathrobe and slippers. They may buy things they don't need but get defensive when asked why they bought them.

What's normal? Making an occasional bad decision or impulsive purchase, but then recognizing and regretting your poor choice.

Withdrawing from Social Activities

People with Alzheimer's may resist going to social functions because they become overwhelmed with all the new faces and conversations swirling around them. They may lose interest in previously enjoyed activities such as football games or Bible study because they can't remember the rules of the game or the points made by the minister. They become flustered when called upon to speak and feel embarrassed when they forget what they were going to say or can't come up with the word they need to complete their sentence. In short, social interactions and activities become mentally draining, embarrassing, and physically exhausting.

What's normal? Sometimes feeling weary of work, family, church, and social obligations, but not because you lose the ability to do them.

—

Retreating to the Past

AD patients will mentally retreat to the time in their life before they had Alzheimer's—when their mother, oldest sister, or favorite dog was still alive, and their wife was a middle-aged brunette. They may not recognize their current house as their home.

What's normal? You should always recognize your spouse and family at their current age and not forget that a loved one or pet is dead. You should always recognize your home.

Changes in Mood and Personality

The mood and personalities of people with Alzheimer's often change. While many remain sweet, some become confused, withdrawn, irritable, suspicious, depressed, accusatory, argumentative, fearful, or fretful. They may become upset, angry, or unreasonable when they are out of their comfort zone. They may throw things like a two-year-old having a temper tantrum. In late stage, they completely withdraw and show little interest in anything.

What's normal? Becoming irritable when a comfortable daily routine gets disrupted.

Interrupted Sleep and Sundown Syndrome

Many Alzheimer's patients catnap throughout the day, but then, at dusk, become restless and start pacing around the house. They refuse to settle down at bedtime and have trouble falling asleep. Others may have no problem falling asleep, but then wake up in the wee hours of the morning feeling restless. Some holler throughout the night. When you try to force the patient to stay awake during the day and go to bed at a reasonable hour, he becomes cranky and unreasonable.

This poorly understood phenomenon of being wide-awake at night is called sundown syndrome. Many caregivers have woken up to find a carton of ice cream melted all over the kitchen counter, drawers emptied, and a general mess to clean up in the morning.

For other patients, nightmares, where the patient wakes up convinced the dream is reality, become common. It may take the caregiver an hour to calm the patient down after a nightmare. In fact, caregiver exhaustion from sleepless nights is one of the major reasons many caregivers feel compelled to admit their loved one to a nursing home.

What's normal? An occasional restless night or the need for fewer hours of sleep as you age. Many seniors find a nap in the afternoon restores their energy enough to complete evening activities. They should still be able to sleep at least four to five hours at night without interruption, as long as they maintain consistent bedtimes and wake up times and don't nod off in their chairs throughout the day.

Incontinence

As the disease progresses into moderate AD, the patient loses the ability to tell when she needs to do bodily functions and will first have urinary incontinence, and in later stages, fecal incontinence.

What's normal? Many older adults struggle with leakage when they sneeze or cough. Many women have trouble getting their pants pulled down fast enough in the bathroom (which is known as urge incontinence). It is ***not*** normal to be unable to sense when you need to urinate or have a bowel movement, however.

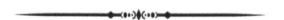

CHAPTER 5

UNDERSTANDING ALZHEIMER'S: Q & A

Dr. Sally Burbank

Do most people become senile when they get old?

While the speed of mental processing may slow as we age, the majority of seniors are not senile. Even at age ninety-five, only half of seniors show definite signs of Alzheimer's disease, and the other half continue to function well. Assuming someone is senile just because they are old is an ungrounded stereotype.

Is getting old the greatest risk factor for Alzheimer's?

Yes, advancing age *is* the greatest risk factor for Alzheimer's disease. Of those currently living with AD, 4 percent are under age sixty-five, 13 percent are sixty-five to seventy-four, 44 percent are seventy-five to eighty-four, and 38 percent are older than eighty-five. Thus, 82 percent of Alzheimer's patients are over the age of seventy-five.

Currently, one in nine people over age sixty-five have Alzheimer's disease, but the risk of developing AD doubles for every five years of life after age 65. By age eighty-five, about one-third of adults have AD. By age ninety-five, half of adults show signs of it.

How long do people with the disease live?

The life expectancy of a person with AD depends on the age of the patient at the time of diagnosis. If they are diagnosed before age seventy, the average length of life is 10.7 years. If they are diagnosed after age ninety, life expectancy is 3.8 years. If all patients with AD are included, the average lifespan is seven years from the time of diagnosis until death.

I couldn't remember the name of a fellow choir member when I ran into him in the grocery store. Does this mean I'm developing early Alzheimer's?

If you recognized the person's face and knew where you knew him from (choir), and the person's name came to you later or sounded familiar when you were told the name, this is not Alzheimer's.

The first warning sign of Alzheimer's disease is repetitive—not occasional—short-term memory loss. You drive to the store to buy milk but can't remember why you went. You repeatedly lose track of where you parked the car, or you get lost driving home from a place you've been to many times. You repeatedly cannot remember where you put your car keys or eyeglasses, and when you find them, you don't remember having put them there. You forget to pay your electric bill. You forget your daughter's birthday, or the details of a phone conversation with your son yesterday. As the disease progresses, you won't even remember that your son called yesterday.

With Alzheimer's, you frequently get confused on what day of the week it is. When you go back to a book you started yesterday, you don't remember the plot or the main characters. You cannot keep up with conversations, and you frequently forget what you were going to say halfway through your story. Family members complain you ask the same questions over and over, and you don't remember the answers they provided five minutes ago. In fact, you don't remember having asked the question at all. Family members accuse you of repeating your same tired stories.

As the disease progresses, you may forget to turn off the stove, feed the dog, or lock up the house at night. You can't remember if you took your morning medications or what you ate for lunch. You don't remember when you last took a shower or bath: Was it yesterday or the day before?

You can see how this presents a very different picture than the usual "senior moments" of normal aging.

Does Alzheimer's only cause short-term memory loss?

No. As the disease progresses, planning and executive abilities are also hindered. Tasks such as following the assembly instructions for a computer desk, subtracting an entry in the checkbook, and staying focused during conversations or board games become a problem.

As AD progresses, the patient uses poor judgment and may buy things she doesn't need and cannot afford. She believes what strangers tell her and can be easily conned. She misplaces things and forgets to record checks or ATM withdrawals in the check registry, leading to bounced checks. Many will insist her dead husband (or sister or cat) is still alive and will become agitated if you try to correct her misinformation.

She may resist bathing and basic hygiene and will show up in public wearing tattered or dirty clothes, often smelling of urine.

As the disease progresses, she can't come up with the name of common objects such as a pencil, penny, or umbrella.

She may have personality changes and become angry, paranoid, unreasonable, or socially withdrawn. She often mixes up her days and nights, catnapping all day and roaming the house at night. She may show up for church on a Monday.

As the disease progresses, patients develop a shuffling gait and become more prone to falls. They develop incontinence.

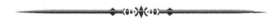

CHAPTER 6

HOW IS ALZHEIMER'S DIAGNOSED?

Dr. Sally Burbank

Objective Tests to Diagnose and Stage AD

The most accurate test currently available to diagnose Alzheimer's disease is a lumbar tap to measure biomarkers in the patient's cerebral spinal fluid. Levels of the biomarker amyloid B1-42 drop by half in AD patients compared to non-demented patients, whereas levels of the biomarkers T-tau and P-tau rise by 200%.

Lumbar tests are rarely used to diagnose AD, however, since many elderly patients have arthritis in their spine or have trouble holding still for a doctor to stick a needle within millimeters of their spinal cord. Most physicians don't perform enough spinal taps to feel competent, and so they are usually done by a neurologist or radiologist. In addition, after a spinal tap is performed, the patient must lie flat for thirty minutes to prevent getting a spinal headache. For all of these reasons, doctors usually try to diagnose Alzheimer's using less invasive tests. Here is a list of the commonly used standardized tests for diagnosing AD:

1. Mini Mental State Exam: The MMSE is considered the gold standard for diagnosing AD. While it is great for monitoring the progression of cognitive decline, I have not personally found it as helpful for picking up the earliest signs of mental decline. The MMSE not only checks a patient's short-term memory, but also checks their ability to follow instructions (such as spell "world" backwards, copy a drawing of two intertwined pentagons, and write a sentence correctly). The patient is asked the year and day of the week and which state he lives in. He is asked to name common items, such as a pen, watch, or chair, and to remember three words. I have a copy of the MMSE on page 53. A perfect score is 30.

Mini-Mental State Examination (MMSE)

Patient's Name: _____   Date: _____

Instructions: *Ask the questions in the order listed. Score one point for each correct response within each question or activity.*

Maximum Score	Patient's Score	Questions
5		"What is the year? Season? Date? Day of the week? Month?"
5		"Where are we now: State? County? Town/city? Hospital? Floor?"
3		The examiner names three unrelated objects clearly and slowly, then asks the patient to name all three of them. The patient's response is used for scoring. The examiner repeats them until patient learns all of them, if possible. Number of trials: _____
5		"I would like you to count backward from 100 by sevens." (93, 86, 79, 72, 65…) Stop after five answers. Alternative: "Spell WORLD backwards." (D-L-R-O-W)
3		"Earlier I told you the names of three things. Can you tell me what those were?"
2		Show the patient two simple objects, such as a wristwatch and a pencil, and ask the patient to name them.
1		"Repeat the phrase: 'No ifs, ands, or buts.'"
3		"Take the paper in your right hand, fold it in half, and put it on the floor." (The examiner gives the patient a piece of blank paper.)
1		"Please read this and do what it says." (Written instruction is "Close your eyes.")
1		"Make up and write a sentence about anything." (This sentence must contain a noun and a verb.)
1		"Please copy this picture." (The examiner gives the patient a blank piece of paper and asks him/her to draw the symbol below. All 10 angles must be present and two must intersect.)
30		TOTAL

(Adapted from Rovner & Folstein, 1987)

The MMSE is scored from 1 to 30 as shown below:

Mini Mental State Exam Scores

30	Perfect Score
29	Still considered normal
26-28	Mild cognitive impairment (but not yet AD)
21-25	Mild Alzheimer's
15-20	Moderate Alzheimer's
10-14	Moderately-Severe Alzheimer's
<10	Severe Alzheimer's

Other common tests to assess memory include:

2. Animal Naming Test: With this test, the patient is asked to name as many animals as he can in one minute. Most adults without dementia can name at least 15 in one minute and 20 in two minutes.

3. The Clock Drawing Test: For this test, the patient has to read instructions and then draw a clock with the hands showing ten minutes after eleven or twenty minutes after eight. Those with AD have difficulty placing the twelve numbers in their proper position and then understanding and executing the instructions to draw the hands of the clock so they point to the proper time. The test is scored on a four-point scale. A score of 3 indicates mild cognitive impairment, and <2 indicates AD.

4. Subtraction Test: This test involves counting backwards by increments of 7, starting with 100. (i.e.100, 93,86,79,72, 65, 58, 51, 44, etc.). I never do this test with those whose educational achievement or IQ is limited, (i.e. those who might have flunked it even when they were teenagers!). A simpler version is to ask the patient to count backwards from 50 by 5's.

5. Three-Word Memorization Test: For this test, state three words, such as Boston, apple, and octopus, and have the patient immediately repeat them back to you. Then inform the patient you will ask him to recall the words in five minutes.

Patients with AD often forget at least one of the three words immediately and need to have them repeated. Repeat the words until the patient can state all three correctly. Then warn the patient you are going to ask him to tell you the words in five minutes. Now distract the patient by doing the Trail-Maker Test or Clock Drawing Test described above. After five minutes, ask the patient to recall the three words. Warning! Many older people will forget one of the three, but they shouldn't forget all three in less than five minutes when they were specifically asked to remember them. When I provide the forgotten word (or words), patients with AD will register no recollection of the forgotten word(s), while those with normal aging or mild cognitive impairment will show recognition of the forgotten word. ("That's right. It was octopus.")

6. Word Pronunciation Test: Ask the patient to repeat back this phrase: "Methodist, Episcopal, Presbyterian." AD patients will stumble over the words or won't be able to remember the three words long enough to repeat them back to you.

7. Mini-Cog Test: Because the Mini-Mental State Exam is time-consuming, many doctors and life insurance companies now rely on the Mini-cog test. This test combines the five-minute three-word memorization test with the clock-drawing test. A perfect score is 5, and any score below 4 is consistent with AD. One point is given for each word remembered, and a perfectly drawn clock with the hands pointing to 11:10 gets a full 2 points. A clock with mistakes gets 0-1 point, depending on how bad the mistakes are.

8. Enhanced Mental Skills Test: This test has an impressive 94% sensitivity for picking up the earliest stages of memory loss and is easy to perform—providing the patient has average reading skills.

Step 1: With a black magic marker, write the following words in bold print on ten individual index cards: CHIMNEY, SALT, HARP, BUTTON, DONKEY, TRAIN, FINGER, FLOWER, RUG, BOOK.

Step 2: Tell the patient you are going to show her ten different words, and you want her to try to remember the words.

Step 3: One at a time, show the patient all ten index cards. Say the word out loud, and then have the patient repeat the word back to you. Go to the next card.

Step 4: After completing all ten words, ask the patient to name every word she can remember. (Don't worry—everybody does badly on this first round!) Record how many words she can remember.

Step 5: Repeat steps 3 and 4 using the same ten cards. Record the number of words the patient remembers with a second try.

Step 6: Repeat steps 3 and 4 a third time, but this time, have the patient use each word in a sentence before advancing to the next card in an effort to jog her memory. Now ask her to name as many of the words as she can remember. Record the number of words remembered after this third try. For most people, the number of words remembered improves dramatically after this third exposure.

Step 7: Now repeat the ten words out loud slowly one more time and tell the patient you are going to ask her to repeat the words in ten minutes. Set a timer for ten minutes, then distract the patient with conversation or another memory test.

Step 8: When the timer goes off, ask the patient to repeat as many of the words as she can remember. Those with no cognitive impairment will remember at least five out of the ten words. Those with mild cognitive impairment will remember four. Alzheimer's patients remember three or fewer words. If it is easier, have the patient write the words she remembers with each trial instead of verbally saying the word out loud.

Step 9: Because test anxiety can sometimes negatively influence even those without memory issues, you can add an additional twist at this point. Pull out ten additional index cards with the following ten words written on them: HOUSE, PEPPER, VIOLIN, ZIPPER, MOUNTAIN, BUS, GOOSE, PENCIL, CHAIR, and TELEVISION.

Shuffle and intersperse the new cards in with the original ten cards. Ask the patient, one card at a time, if the word is one of the original ten words. Patients without AD have no trouble at all separating the ten original words from the newly introduced words. Those with AD will be unsure or will just guess.

9. The Trail-Maker Test: This is a more challenging test and is timed. The patient must draw a continuous line alternating from number to letter and back to a number, starting with 1-A and progressing upward to 12-L. (See sample below.) When a patient loses the ability to do this test correctly in under two minutes, he should give up his driver's license. If he only makes one or two mistakes and can then find and correct them, the cognitive function is still intact enough to drive.

Trail Making (Part B)

Patient's Name: _____   Date: _____

A correctly executed Trail-Maker test.

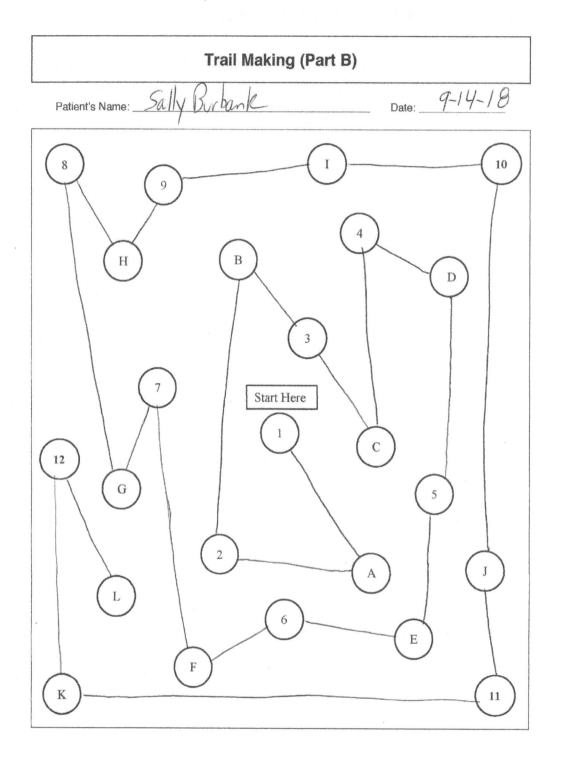

CHAPTER 7

REACTIONS TO THE DIAGNOSIS
Sue Bell

Since there is no known cure for Alzheimer's disease, the diagnosis is devastating—both to patients and their families. When Ray was confronted with the diagnosis, his first response was, "Sue, I'm afraid I'll forget your name." This was a very difficult moment for both of us. I assured him it would be okay, but truthfully, I was as upset as he was.

As a caregiver, there are many decisions that must be made and many unknowns to face. There will be times when you're convinced the doctor was wrong, and you want to deny the diagnosis, especially in the early stage when the patient will have good days and seem relatively fine. Then, day-by-day, as the patient declines and there are fewer good days, you quietly accept the diagnosis, and feel less panicky and more capable of handling the situation.

Here are some of the reactions expressed when patients were informed they had Alzheimer's:

- Emily D., when asked how she was doing, informed me, "I think I have that awful disease. You know, the one where you can't remember things."

- Caroline M. broke down in tears and said, "I don't want to face this."

- Mary C. reported that when the doctor told her husband he wasn't allowed to drive because he had moderate-stage Alzheimer's, he got angry and called the doctor a quack. "That doctor doesn't know what he's talking about." He refused to take the medication the doctor prescribed and insisted there was nothing wrong with him.

- Sylvia P. said when the doctor told her husband he had Alzheimer's and wasn't allowed to drive anymore, he said nothing. When they got home, he laid his keys in a drawer and never tried to drive again. He also never talked about it.

- Phyllis M.'s husband heard the diagnosis and snapped, "That doctor doesn't run this house, I do, so I don't care what he says."

- John F. acted like he never heard the diagnosis. Since he was already in a later stage, he probably had forgotten everything the doctor said by the time he reached home.

- One common response: "Promise me you won't put me in a nursing home."

- Another common response is denial: "Everybody's memory declines as they get older," or "I never did have a good memory," or "It's just a senior moment."

- "Why me? What did I do to deserve this?"

- "This is not what I had planned for our golden years."

- "Will we have the finances to survive this?"

- "Will my wife divorce me?"

Dealing with Shame
Dr. Sally Burbank

Many of my older patients and their spouses seem to feel shame or embarrassment when diagnosed with AD and don't want anyone to know. I have been amazed how many caregivers keep their loved one cloistered in the house and avoid telling anyone their husband or wife has dementia. Many elders have shared the news to me in a whisper voice and asked me not to tell anyone—as though a diagnosis of AD is shameful. Since AD is a disease and not a moral failing, I have never understood the stigma that is still rampant in the general public with a diagnosis of Alzheimer's. I try to educate my patients and their caregivers that Alzheimer's is a medical condition and nothing to be ashamed of.

Common reactions to the diagnosis:

- "You must be mistaken; she couldn't have Alzheimer's."
- "Will my spouse/kids put me in a nursing home and forget about me?"
- "I don't want to be a burden to my family."
- "I'd rather be dead than lose my mind."
- "Isn't there something you can do to keep me from getting worse?"
- "What about that new supplement I heard about on TV—the one made from jellyfish?"
- "His memory is better than mine. He still knows all the state capitols."
- "Mom is just grieving. After all, Dad only died a year ago."

- "He's been under tremendous stress lately. That's all it is."

Once the diagnosis sinks in, caregivers have worries, too:

- "I don't want to be a nurse."
- "I'm ashamed to have people know. George was always so smart."
- "How long before he doesn't know who I am anymore?"
- "I feel so alone. I'm afraid to face this."
- "Will I be able to handle him? What if he becomes violent?"
- "Surely medicine will help."
- "My life is over. I'll never get to enjoy my golden years."
- "I'll be stuck caretaking someone who won't even know who I am. What's in this for me?"
- "I don't want to deal with this—it's overwhelming."
- "I resent having to take care of him. He wasn't even a faithful husband."
- "What if I don't have what it takes to care for someone with no memory? Will I have the patience and stamina to deal with this?"

- "She's only sixty-two. I thought Alzheimer's was a disease of old people."
- "How am I going to competently care for my husband and kids if I'm having to care of Dad?"

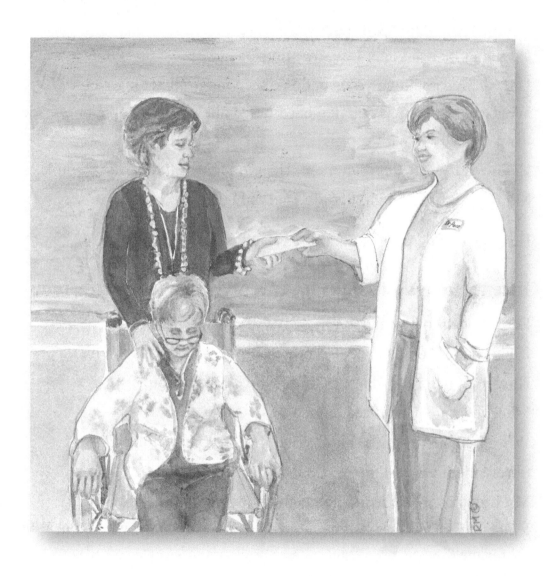

CHAPTER 8

STAGES OF ALZHEIMER'S
Dr. Sally Burbank

Physicians often divide Alzheimer's disease into three stages: early, middle, and late. In reality, the three stages overlap, but the general trend is a gradual downward trajectory. Here are the typical symptoms of each stage:

Early-stage Alzheimer's

Early-stage Alzheimer's disease usually goes undiagnosed. Caregivers dismiss the occasional memory lapses as simple aging or a "senior moment." Fatigue or stress is often blamed. Doctors may try to alleviate your fears by insisting Mom's memory issues are merely side effects of her medications—especially her pain, sleep, and incontinence pills. Medical conditions that cause chronic pain, depression, or insufficient sleep make easy scapegoats for memory issues because these conditions *do* exacerbate difficulty with memory. Grieving the loss of a spouse will absolutely contributes to cognitive issues.

Thus, diagnosing AD in its earliest stage can be tricky.

Another cause for a delay in diagnosing AD early is that the patient has good and bad days. Just when you are convinced Mom has early Alzheimer's, she will turn around and have an on-target day where she seems completely normal. Perhaps because we psychologically don't *want* Mom to have AD, we dismiss our fears and choose to think the on-target days are the norm, and the memory-challenged days are a fluke. With time, however, when there are fewer on-target days and more off-target days, the truth becomes harder to ignore.

The symptoms of early AD are most pronounced when the patient is tired, such as at bedtime or after a draining social event. In short, Mom's cognitive reserve gets depleted, and she can no longer compensate. Thus, she may seem confused one day and fine the next morning after a night of sleep.

In hindsight, the signs of early AD will become obvious, but for the reasons stated above, AD usually isn't formally diagnosed until the middle stage when short-term memory lapses become the norm.

Once the diagnosis of AD is made, many of the troublesome changes you have been observing in your loved one will make sense. As the disease progresses, the symptoms listed below will increase in frequency and severity:

- **Short-term memory loss.** Patients may remember exact details of events from their childhood but not something you told them yesterday. They forget whether they've taken their morning medications or what they ate for supper last night. They forget birthdays or a scheduled doctor's appointment.

- **Difficulty with word finding.** Patients repeatedly cannot come up with the correct word in a conversation and will have to describe what they are trying to say. For example; "That thing that cleans the carpet," instead of vacuum, or "That thing that unclogs the toilet," instead of plunger.

- **Difficulty driving.** Even when driving in familiar locations, they take wrong turns or fail to yield to oncoming traffic when turning left. They may not stop and look at yield signs. Getting lost is aggravated after dark when familiar road cues become less obvious.

- **Poor financial decisions.** They may buy things they don't need, especially from TV advertisers or scammers. Their pantry may have fifteen cans of beef stew because they don't remember they stocked up on beef stew last week.

- **Defensiveness.** Patients become irritable and defensive if you bring up their bounced checks, memory lapses, or concerns that they shouldn't be driving.

- **Losing focus in a conversation.** They lose their train of thought in a conversation and can't finish their story or make the point they wanted to make.

- **Repetition.** They repeat their stories, questions, and comments.

- **Inability to retain what they read.** They can't remember the characters or plot of a book they started yesterday. Consequently, as AD progresses, previously avid readers find reading novels frustrating. They cannot retain what they read in the morning newspaper.

Middle-stage Alzheimer's

In the middle stage, the symptoms listed above become more pronounced and disrupt life on a daily basis. The cognitive issues are no longer merely annoying, they become dangerous, especially if the patient is still trying to live alone or drive. They now require more diligent daily oversight.

The middle stage lasts for several years and includes:

- **Forgetting.** AD patients confuse and forget the names, faces, birthdays, and phone numbers of friends and family members. They forget their own address, social security number, and phone number.

- **Overreactive and volatile emotional reactions.** Simple problems, such as the inability to complete a task or a change in plans, can trigger a histrionic or calamitous emotional reaction. Patients may stubbornly refuse to go to the doctor's office one day but be docile the next. They may throw their food or act out in childish ways. Erratic mood swings become common, so the caregiver may feel she must capitulate to the patient's every whim to avoid a blow-up or catastrophic reaction.

- **Living in the past.** The patient may claim he needs to milk the cows or tend to the cattle even though the cows were sold years earlier. Some women will think dolls are living babies that need care. Patients may mentally freeze the age of their grandchildren to when they were babies or very young. They may not grasp that the adult visiting them *is* their grandchild now grown up, because the concept of aging doesn't register. A man may not grasp that the gray-haired lady who cares for him is his spouse of fifty years. He may insist she is an imposter—or his mother.

- **Suspiciousness.** Because patients can't remember where they left something or where they spent their money, they often accuse spouses, children, nurses, or visitors of stealing.

- **Erratic sleep cycles.** Patients may nod off in their chair during the day, then roam the house at night. They may become agitated after sundown.

- **Ignoring personal hygiene.** Because they can't remember when they last took a bath or shower, patients may go weeks without one if family members don't intervene. They may need supervision to ensure they choose weather-appropriate and clean clothing. If left to their own devices, many seem content to wear the same frayed and food-stained clothes for days on end. Some become frightened by running water, adding to the difficulty of bathing and showering. Many resist bathing. They forget how to brush their teeth, shampoo and style their hair, put on makeup, or shave. Unless they wear a large bib when eating, they spill food all over their clothes and make a mess of their eating space.

- **Inability to complete complex tasks.** Driving, banking, shopping, cooking meals, doing laundry, planning and executing social events—all will have to be taken over or supervised by a caregiver.

- **Communication becomes more challenging.** Patients have ever-increasing difficulty finding the appropriate words to complete their sentences or to articulate what they want. They have problems understanding more than simple, one-step directions, and you may need to demonstrate with hand gestures what you want them to do. They forget what they were going to say in the middle of a sentence. They can't stay focused in a conversation because they forget what you said two minutes ago. They may slur their speech when they are tired. When conversations become too challenging or frustrating, they give up or just repeat the same statement or question over and over. They may become irritable when frustrated or when they feel left out.

- **Repetition.** They repeat comments, questions, or stories until you want to scream. Examples include: "Whose house is this?", "I want to go home.", "Who are you?", "Where is my wife?", or "Where is my mother?" They often appear lost and afraid. One Alzheimer's patient informed me seven times during his annual exam, "My mother lived to be 104."

- **Isolation or progressive muteness.** Because staying focused in conversations becomes difficult, they begin to isolate themselves and prefer to stay home. Or, they may go to the family reunion and say little or nothing. Large social gatherings become bewildering if the trusted caregiver isn't at their side. They may resist attending family social events, senior citizen centers, or church functions because interacting with others is frustrating, humiliating, and overwhelming. As they near the late stage, they may quit talking altogether, or just mouth monosyllables or repetitive short phrases.

- **Simple tasks become difficult.** As the middle stage progresses to the late stage, even simple tasks become impossible. Tasks they could perform in the early and middle stage—using the remote control, setting the table, loading the dishwasher, doing a load of laundry, buttoning a shirt properly, reading the paper— now prove to be too difficult. They may try to use the remote control as a phone receiver or put the milk in the pantry instead of the refrigerator. They may run a load of laundry without detergent or pour in half a bottle of detergent. They will forget the steaming vegetables on the stove until the water has boiled out and the smoke detector goes off. Even then, some won't register what the loud noise means—it only frightens them.

- **Not recognizing themselves or family members in pictures.** They may revert to thinking their childhood home is their real home. They may confuse their wife with their mother or their husband with their father.

- **Difficulty eating with a fork and knife.** They may have to use large handgrip utensils, have their food cut up for them, or eat finger foods.

- **Difficulty going to the bathroom independently.** They may go to the bathroom in inappropriate places such as an umbrella holder. They may use too much toilet paper or forget to flush. When they reach end stage, they lose the ability to know they need to go and will have complete urinary and fecal incontinence.

- **Loss of temperature awareness.** They may seem clueless that they are outside in freezing weather without a coat. They may turn up the thermostat to 90 degrees. They may not feel pain appropriately.

- **Enjoyment of music.** They often enjoy music from the decade when they were teenagers or young adults. Music may bring back emotions and memories of a more pleasant time in their lives. It also tends to calm and distract them when they are agitated.

- **Obsession with dead pets or family members.** Many AD patients can't remember that their mother, sister, or favorite pet is dead. They may repeatedly call for a cat or dog that died three years ago or insist they want to call their dead sister on the phone. When informed the pet or loved one is dead, they become upset and insist you are wrong.

- **Personality change.** Their personality may change until they seem to be just a shell of who they used to be. The hardest part of AD is witnessing an intelligent, warm, funny loved one slowly disintegrate into someone who is frightened, confused, and progressively mute.

- **Getting lost and wandering off.** If they are physically healthy, patients may wander off when your back is turned or when you are taking a shower. They may get lost in a restaurant after leaving the bathroom, as they don't remember where your table is or maybe even who you are. They may walk to the mailbox and then get confused and wander in the wrong direction because they don't recognize the house.

Late-stage Alzheimer's

By late-stage AD, the patient becomes dependent on caregivers for even the most basic of daily living tasks. If the caregiver doesn't solicit help, this stage will be exhausting. Thankfully, some things are easier in this stage. Patients sleep up to eighteen hours per day, which frees up time to get chores done or to indulge in a favorite hobby. Patients often become more docile and cooperative and less prone to roaming off and getting lost. They are most content to be at home with a predictable routine.

In late stage, though they no longer converse much, they still need and crave affection. Pat their arms, hold their hands, smile, and continue to talk to them in a calm, loving voice, even when they don't seem to understand your words. They will register your tone of voice and your facial expression. You will be the center of their world as they become dependent on you for their every need. It is a big responsibility to help someone through this phase, but it doesn't last forever.

End-stage Alzheimer's

What should I expect when the disease reaches end-stage?

- **Round-the-clock care.** The patient will need twenty-four-hour care, and you may need help with feeding, meds, bathing, laundry, shopping, paying bills, yard work, and housework.

- **Weight loss.** The patient will lose weight, even though you are offering nutritious meals, because she is sleeping most of the time. As she spends more time sleeping, her muscles atrophy. Even when awake, she won't eat much—because her appetite dwindles—and you won't be able to make her eat. She will seem unaware whether she is hungry or not, or, if she is hungry, she won't be able to find the words to tell you. Most have to be spoon fed or shown how to scoop up food with a spoon at every meal.

- **Inability to recognize self in a picture or mirror.** The patient may seem to recognize someone but have no knowledge of who the person is or her connection to the person. One patient, when asked to find himself in a family photo, pointed to his son who looked like a younger version of himself. When asked who the older gentleman standing next to his son was, he replied, "I have no idea." (He was the older gentleman.)

- **Inability to communicate needs.** She will become progressively more inarticulate and mute, requiring a guessing game to know what she wants. She may frequently moan and groan. Hand gestures or pictures may aide in communicating.

- **Rituals.** He may resort to repetitive actions, such as shredding paper, rocking, pacing, or wringing his hands when agitated.

- **Hallucinations.** The patient may claim to see and communicate with dead relatives or pets. She may pick up things that are not visible to anyone else, suggesting visual hallucinations. She may talk to stuffed animals or dolls as though they are alive. One AD patient, a retired minister who had preached at many funerals, had a wind-up toy monkey that would walk across the floor. The pastor got many hours of enjoyment talking to and playing with his toy monkey. One day, the monkey's arm fell off. The pastor tried to put the arm back in its socket numerous times, but when the arm wouldn't stay, he took out his handkerchief, carefully wrapped up the monkey, and placed it gently on a shelf. He never tried to take the monkey back down from the shelf. It was as if he had buried his toy monkey.

- **Excessive sleeping.** The patient may sleep up to 20 hours a day.

- **Getting lost.** He may get lost *even in his own home*. You may have to lead him to his bedroom, the bathroom, or the living room.

- **Assistance with all personal hygiene.** She can no longer independently bathe, brush her hair or teeth, put on clothes and shoes, button a blouse or zip up pants. He will no longer remember how to shave.

- **Disinterest in life.** She will lose interest in her surroundings and what's going on in the world, including family events. Even activities that used to pique her interest hold no appeal. She may do little more than eat and sleep and stare into space.

- **Difficulty with swallowing.** He may forget to swallow and may squirrel away food in his cheeks. Choking becomes a potential hazard.

- **Bathroom issues.** She may forget how to use the bathroom and will lose control over her bowels and bladder, which suggests that even the most basic of physiological cues from the body to the brain are gone. Or, if it does register, she may be unable to articulate the need or find her way to the bathroom.

- **Nightmares.** He may moan, groan, or holler in his sleep, which suggests he is having a nightmare.

- **Seizures.** Thankfully, seizures are rare.

- **Inability to wake up.** She may sleep with her eyes half-opened, and she may be hard to arouse.

- **Falling out of beds or chairs.** Loss of posture and strength become common. He may lose his ability to sit upright. Propping up with pillows can help if you have a wheelchair with a seatbelt. In cars, seat belts and shoulder harnesses do the trick.

- **Eating inappropriate things.** Pencil erasers, coins, buttons, nuts, or cherry pits can all pose choking hazards.

- **Falls and difficulty with walking.** Incidents of falls and hip fractures are quadrupled in patients with late-stage Alzheimer's. Walking becomes slow and shuffling. By the end stage, she may become largely bed bound.

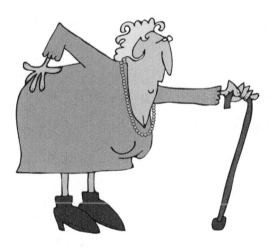

CHAPTER 9

FUNCTIONAL ASSESSMENT AND STAGING
Dr. Sally Burbank

The spouses and children of AD patients often want to know how advanced their loved one's AD is and what to expect next. Barry Reisberg developed a Functional Assessment Staging Tool (FAST) to assist families in grading their loved one's condition. Here are the major benchmarks:

No Cognitive Decline

- No obvious neurological deficits are perceived by patient or family.
- MMSE score is 29-30. (Perfect score is 30.)

Mild Cognitive Decline (Age-Related Memory Impairment)

- Patient forgets where she puts famgiliar objects such as keys, glasses, or remote control.
- Patient suffers occasional inability to come up with a word she wanted to say or the name of a person she knows well.
- MMSE score is 26-28.
- Progresses to dementia 60 percent of the time.

Very Early Dementia (Lasts up to seven years)

- Co-workers and family now notice an increasing number of mistakes and a general forgetfulness in the patient.

- Patient has difficulty navigating to new locations without getting lost, even if provided with a map or written instructions.

- Patient has decreased ability to stay organized. Must write everything down and can no longer rely on memory alone to function.

- Patient forgets appointments and previous conversations.

- Patient repeats stories and questions.

- Patient's word-finding deficit becomes obvious to others.

- MMSE score is 23-25, which shows an objective deficit.

Mild Dementia/Early Dementia (Lasts two years on average)

- Patient shows decreased ability to handle complex tasks such as planning, shopping for, and executing a dinner party; paying bills on time; taking out the trash or recycling on the correct day without being reminded.

- Patient finds counting money a challenge and cannot subtract correctly in the checkbook.

- Patient arrives at church or doctor's appointment late or on the wrong day.

- Patient still knows the names and faces of family members and close friends and can travel to familiar places like the grocery store and church without getting lost.

- Patient can no longer can count backwards from 100 by 7's.

- MMSE score is 20-22.

Moderate Dementia (Lasts 1.5 years on average)

- Patient requires help in selecting clothes appropriate for the occasion and weather conditions.

- Patient is still able to dress herself, use toilet, and eat independently.

- Patient may not remember her home address, phone number, day of the week, college alma mater, or names of grandchildren, but still knows who she is and the names of her spouse and children.

- Patient struggles with counting backward from 40 by 4's and can no longer retain what she reads.
- MMSE score is 18-19

Moderately Severe Dementia (Lasts 2.5 years, on average)

- Patient requires assistance with putting on clothes properly (buttons, shoes, shoelaces, etc.).
- Patient is unable to bathe or shower independently. She cannot adjust water temperature or remember when she last took a bath.
- Patient can't handle the mechanics of toileting properly. She doesn't remember to flush or wipe. He doesn't remember to zip up his fly.
- Urinary, and then fecal incontinence become increasingly common.
- Patient begins to forget the names and faces of spouse and children, but often still knows her own name.
- Patient has trouble counting backwards from 10 or reciting the alphabet.

As things progress toward severe dementia, the patient may:

- Become delusional and think spouse is an imposter.
- Talk to imaginary figures, dolls, or to her own image in the mirror.
- Pace, sundown, or engage in obsessive rituals like cleaning or ripping paper.
- Become violent when agitated.
- Forget what she is told within five minutes and consequently, she repeats her questions repetitively. Patient is unable to retain recent news events seen on TV or the plot and characters of television programs or books.
- MMSE score is usually less than 15 but ranges up to 17.

Severe Dementia (Lasts 2.5 years on average)

- Patient's ability to speak is now reduced to six or fewer different words in the course of an extended conversation or day. This will progress downward until speech is limited to a single intelligible word or phrase over the course of a day.

- Patient may repeat a single word or phrase over and over. Speech will decline further until she can only communicate with grunts, moans, or unintelligible words.

- Patient gets lost in her own home and gradually becomes unable to walk without assistance.

- Patient may have to be shown how to hold a spoon to scoop up food at mealtime.

- Patient will lose weight.

- MMSE score is less than 10, (but most can't complete the test at all).

End-Stage Dementia (Only lasts a few months)

- Patient is unable to eat, talk, walk, or do anything independently. Rarely smiles or reacts.

- Patient can no longer sit in a chair without armrests without falling forward.

- Patient must be spoon fed. She may frequently choke, as she will forget how to swallow and will squirrel food away in her cheeks.

- Patient suffers from complete incontinence of bowels and bladder.

- Patient sleeps up to 20 hours per day.

- Patient is bed-bound.

- Patient usually dies from aspiration pneumonia, choking, kidney infection, or kidney failure due to dehydration.

PART II

CARING FOR ALZHEIMER'S PATIENTS

CHAPTER 10

—◆◦‹•›◦✦◦‹•›◦◆—

WORLD OF EMOTIONS
Sue Bell

Emotions

Farewell to the world of reason, and welcome to the world of emotions.

As AD patients' minds deteriorate, their emotional responses become heightened. They now function through their senses instead of their minds, navigating through life by relying on what they see, hear, smell, taste, and feel. They still recognize a smiling face as being happy, and they enjoy hearing a favorite song or hymn. Until the late stage, they enjoy a tasty piece of chocolate cake or apple pie, as well as the smell of lilacs and apple blossoms, though the sense of smell declines in AD. The giggle of a baby or the beauty of a favorite mountain vista may trigger pleasant memories and bring joy. Memories with an emotion attached to it—fear, anger, or joy—are more likely to be retained because memories with emotions tap into additional parts of the brain.

Since they cannot plan for the future, Alzheimer's patients live in the moment, enjoying the signals their senses provide.

<u>Sight</u>: Ray had always been an avid golfer. Once his AD became severe, he could no longer talk. Nevertheless, he would get excited every time I drove by the golf course, as it clearly triggered pleasant memories. I would let him ride around in a golf cart and enjoy the fresh air and sunshine. It always made him smile, even though he couldn't voice his feelings.

<u>Sound</u>: One time, when Ray was at his daughter's birthday party, he suddenly joined us in singing "Happy Birthday," even though he hadn't spoken in weeks. The whole family watched in amazement. Music especially spurs

—

memories. Many can sing songs they knew as a child even into the later stages of AD. My mother could join me in singing, "She'll Be Coming 'Round the Mountain" and "Jesus Loves Me" long after she stopped talking.

Lily R. heard her husband's voice as he talked to someone in the hall outside her nursing home room. She told the nurse, "That's my husband in the hall." When he entered her room, however, she looked at him with a quizzical expression and asked, "Who are you?" She had recognized his voice, but not his face!

Familiar Activities: Karen N. hired someone to sit with her father at night. The young man later told her that the father wanted to play checkers, though he probably hadn't played in forty years. "He beat me every single game, and I wasn't letting him win!"

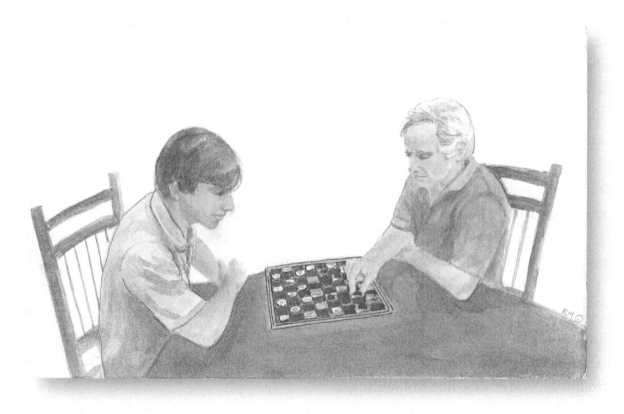

Smells: Gloria B. frequently refused to eat, so her children started bringing her into the kitchen when they cooked. They purposely seasoned the food with her favorite herbs and spices: garlic, oregano, cinammon, and ginger. Before long, her mouth would water, and she would ask to try some of the food. Gloria said this worked every time.

In addition to their senses, patients rely on facial expressions and the tone of their caregiver's voice to interpret if all is well.

AD patients will occasionally have moments of amazing clarity. It is difficult to determine what triggers these precious moments, or if they will ever happen again, so cherish them when they happen.

Unfortunately, there are times when nothing works. One gentleman was convinced his wife had died. He kept asking for her by name, even though she was sitting with him in the room. He just couldn't grasp that she was his wife, even when she showed him photos of the two of them together. He couldn't recognize her or himself in the photos. Her voice, the smell of her perfume, her long-worn red apron and wooly winter coat—none of these triggered a memory.

Your reactions, attitudes, and emotions will signal to the patient how to react. If you are happy, she will be happy. If you are angry or frustrated, she will feel your tension and react in an agitated manner. In short, AD patients don't feel secure if the caregiver is upset.

Ray constantly watched my face to see my reaction to things. If I smiled, he smiled. If someone was angry, he detected it and became upset. I'll never forget one harrowing experience:

A gentleman who had done some mowing for us came to our house to be paid. He sat down at the kitchen table to visit with us. Our visitor was extremely upset because his teenaged daughter had grabbed his glasses in a fit of rage and stomped on them. He spoke about the incident with an agitated voice. I was listening intently, probably with a horrified expression on my face. As the man shared his story, he made angry gestures with his hands, and his voice grew louder. Suddenly, Ray got up and left the room. He came back with a raised golf club, ready to clobber the man in an effort to protect me!

Obviously, Ray could not understand what the man and I were discussing. He could only register the man's angry voice and hand gestures. Thinking the man was angry with us, he felt threatened. I jumped up and gently took the golf club from Ray while smiling and patting him on the shoulder. I explained, in a reassuring voice, that I was fine. He calmed down when he saw I was not angry or upset.

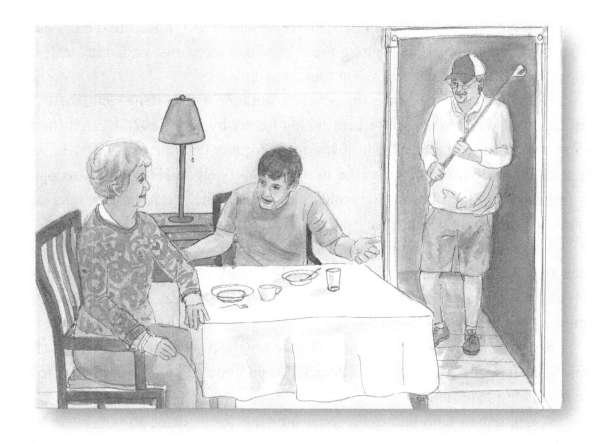

My mother, who also suffered from dementia, had a sitter who sometimes fussed at her. At breakfast one morning, the sitter scolded mother for not eating enough breakfast. Mother reacted by picking up her mug of coffee and flinging it into the woman's face. "I've never done anything to you," Mother hissed. She had interpreted the sitter's admonishing words and displeased facial expression as anger. Like toddlers, AD patients can act impulsively when they feel threatened or upset.

Since AD patients will mirror back the emotions they see written on your face, make a point to smile and gently touch their shoulder or hand. This small act reassures them and works wonders. If you don't feel like smiling, fake it! Here's why:

Imagine being suddenly plunked into a strange country where you don't speak the language or even know where you are. If the person across from you smiles, pats your shoulder, and speaks in a soothing tone, you will interpret all is well, even though you don't have a clue what is being said. But what if the stranger is scowling or shouting at you with an upraised fist? Your interpretation? *I don't like this place. I don't feel safe.* That is what life is like for an Alzheimer's patient. He will reach a point when he won't remember who his caregiver is or the gist of the conversation swirling around him. He must rely on the caregiver's facial expressions and tone of voice to interpret if things are okay.

We instinctively know how to treat babies. Since they don't understand our words, we smile, coo, and cuddle them to make them feel secure. We can reassure our AD patient using the same soothing behaviors. Give hugs and pat their arm or shoulder. Hold their hand and smile. Speak in a pleasant tone and use simple words.

Use hand gestures to demonstrate what you want them to do. As they progress into later stages, they may not understand the words, "Eat your oatmeal," but they will recognize hand gestures of scooping up food and bringing it to their mouth. They can watch you demonstrate how to bring a toothbrush to their mouth and brush.

In summary, AD patients have mirror-image behavior. They see the world through your reactions, and they will react based on your tone of voice, gestures, and facial expressions.

Should I Correct Misinformation?

Dr. Sally Burbank and Sue Bell

Due to their damaged brains, the memories of AD patients are often inaccurate. As a consequence, they may say things that are just plain wrong. Should

---

you correct the patient? Research shows arguing with a patient or correcting misinformation will not change the AD patient's perception of reality. If anything, it will likely upset her. Instead, let it go, (unless having accurate information is crucial for safety reasons). Keep in mind, the patient won't remember the conversation in ten minutes anyway. Worse, she may insist you are lying to her.

Examples of Dealing with a Confused Patient

- When Betty D.'s daughter, Valerie, and sixteen-year-old grandson, Jason, came for a visit, Betty asked where baby Jason was. Valerie pointed to Jason and explained that "baby Jason" was now all grown up. Throughout the visit, however, Betty would repeat her same tiresome question, "Where's baby Jason?" Valerie explained—repeatedly—that Jason was no longer a baby. The fifth time Betty asked, "Where's baby Jason?" Jason told his Granny that a neighbor was watching the baby, so they could come for a visit. Betty stopped asking.

- Margaret M.'s mind had reverted back to the years when her daughter, Amy, now a married mother living in another state, was in high school. When it was bedtime, Margaret fretted that something terrible had happened to Amy since she hadn't come home from school and hadn't called to say where she was. Her caregiver husband, John, knew from past experience that telling Margaret her daughter was now a thirty-two-year-old mother living in Dallas would do no good. In fact, it would only agitate her. She would accuse him of lying or keeping Amy's whereabouts from her. As Margaret paced the living room, John knew he had to do something to relieve her anxiety, so he thumped his forehead and told her, "Oh, I forgot to tell you. Amy called, and she is spending the night at a friend's house. I meant to tell you." After Margaret bawled him out for not remembering to tell her, John apologized and then distracted her with, "Let's go make a nice warm cup of tea, shall we?" Worries relieved, Margaret quit fretting. John rationalized his white lie by telling himself that Amy was indeed spending the night with a friend— her husband!

• Sometimes humor can help, as Carol B. discovered. Carol's mother would often say, "I want to call Sara" (her deceased sister). Carol would inform her, "Sara is in heaven. Do you have God's phone number?" Her mother would laugh and call her silly.

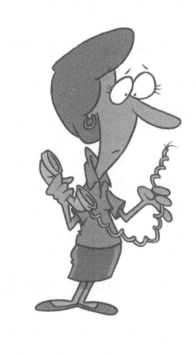

CHAPTER 11

CAREGIVING ESSENTIALS
Sue Bell and Dr. Sally Burbank

Caregiving Options

Approximately ten million Alzheimer's patients in the United States are cared for at home by family, and millions more are cared for in nursing homes or memory care facilities.

When no healthy spouse is available to care for a patient in the early stages, some may be able to live alone in their home as long as someone checks in on them daily. Once a patient reaches the moderate stage, however, independent living is no longer an option, and alternative arrangements must be made.

Possible Caregiving Arrangements

- A caregiver or family member moves into the patient's house. If the patient has multiple children, they can alternate staying with Mom or Dad any given day or night. Or, one can be the primary caregiver while the other siblings provide back up when the main caregiver needs a break or has an appointment.

- The patient moves into the home of a relative or friend.

- The patient goes to an assisted living facility that transitions into a nursing home as the patient's condition worsens.

- The patient goes to an adult daycare during the workday and lives with the family at night and on weekends.

- The patient goes to a specialized memory care facility.

Family Choices

- The Jones family had four adult children. The siblings alternated taking Mom into their home for two weeks at a time. That way, the main care was divided with each child providing care for two weeks every two months. This arrangement worked for three or four years. When the mother became too frail to move from house to house, the children placed her in a nursing home for the last year of her life. They took turns visiting her daily to ensure she received good care.

- The Hall family kept their mother in her own home by having the children and grandchildren coordinate who would stay with her each night. Relying on multiple caregivers requires careful organization and reliability.

- Marge J. had three adult children who lived nearby. Two had good jobs and nice homes, but one daughter, Tina, had recently divorced, had three children, no job, and a tiny rented apartment she could barely afford. The two financially well-off siblings worked it out for Tina to move into their mother's home and care for Mom until she died. She lived off their mother's Social security and pension, and when Mother died, Tina got to keep the house and the remaining equity in the estate. This was a win-win for everyone, as Mother was able to stay in her home with a loving caregiver until the end, and Tina had a full-time job and ended up with a paid-for home and small nest egg. Tina's living expenses were adequately covered by her mother's monthly Social Security checks, retirement accounts, and the life insurance money Mom received when her husband died.

- Sarah D., a retired teacher whose husband had AD, decided to move them both into an assisted living facility. Despite her husband's moderately severe condition, they were accepted into the facility because the wife was able to provide basic care. Sarah gave her husband his medicines and took care of his personal needs, while the facility provided meals, social interaction, laundry services, and transportation to the grocery and doctor's office. The front desk was also alerted to watch for her husband should he ever try to roam the halls at night while Sarah was asleep.

- Jack S. gave his daughter enough money to build a small addition to her home in case it was ever needed for himself or his wife.

- Mary L. had a full-time job. She discovered her mother was no longer safe living alone after her mother left a pot of macaroni cooking on the stove long after the water boiled out. Mother had ignored the smoke detector alarm because she didn't know what it meant. Mary enrolled her mother in an adult daycare, picked her up after work, and cared for her in her home on nights and weekends.

- Margaret M. chose to put her mother in an excellent memory care facility so that her mother could benefit from all the AD-appropriate activities and social interactions that the center provided. Margaret felt overwhelmed at the prospect of caring for her mother by herself and felt more secure knowing her mother was being looked after by a staff experienced with Alzheimer's patients. Margaret visited her mother regularly, so she wouldn't feel abandoned.

- In my situation, I retired from my job so that I could care for my husband, Ray, at home. Occasionally, a family member or a sitter helped me. I looked at caregiving as my new job, as it would have been very costly to put him in a nursing home. Also, I wanted him to stay at home and enjoy our yard. Ray had worked hard his whole life and had diligently saved money for retirement. Before he was diagnosed, we had discussed our wishes if either of us became incapacitated. We both wanted to stay at home, as long as it was financially and physically possible. I solved problems as they came up and tried to enjoy life at each stage.

Some people have no choice but to put their loved one in a nursing home. They may have full-time jobs to support their own families and may not have an extra bedroom or the finances to hire a full-time sitter. In rural areas, there may not be an adult daycare or competent sitter available. The patient may have caregiving needs that cannot be met at home, especially if the patient is obese, violent, or impossible to deal with. Sometimes, the relationship between the AD patient and child is so fractured or volatile they simply cannot live together without wanting to kill each other! Some AD patients have no children to care for them, or the children are incapable or unwilling to care for a parent with dementia. Some lack the nurturing personality and patience required to competently care for someone who may ask the same question twenty times or who may wander off and get lost. At least in a nursing home or memory care center, the patient will be safe and cared for by trained personnel. Another benefit? Memory care facilities provide stimulating activities and the opportunity to socialize.

Daycare centers make it possible to keep Mom in your home at night and on weekends, but still keep her safe and protected while you are at work. Plus, daycare is much cheaper than a nursing home or memory care center. The downside? The caregiver must get Mom bathed, dressed, fed, and transported to the daycare facility every morning and then ensure she is picked up before the center closes. Since some AD patients become stubborn or uncooperative when rushed, this can make getting Mom to the daycare and you to your job on time a daily challenge! Adult daycare centers are usually open weekdays only, so you will need to be responsible for Mom's care every weekend. Some cities have respite care centers, which allow for the occasion weekend off, but they are expensive and not covered by Medicare. Adult daycares are also usually not covered by Medicare or Medicaid.

If the patient is not a homeowner and has no life savings or income, except for social security, the nursing home option may actually be cheaper than adult daycare. Why? If a patient is poor, Medicaid covers nursing home costs.

Assisted living programs are helpful in early AD when the patient is still able to handle her own bathing, dental hygiene, and dressing, but as the patient progresses to the moderately severe stage and full dependency, assisted living programs are not equipped to handle these demands (unless they have a progressive program that evolves into a full Alzheimer's nursing home unit). Assisted living programs are expensive, and over the years I have found many of my middle-income and lower-income patients cannot afford them.

Nursing Homes: A Financial Drain

Unless your loved one has no savings, home, or assets—and thereby qualifies for Medicaid—admitting them into a nursing home is very costly. In 2017, the national average topped $228 per day—which adds up to a whopping $83,220 per year. The prices vary by state and by facility. In Tennessee, the average yearly cost is $70,000. At these astronomical prices, elderly patients can run through their life's savings quickly.

Does Medicare cover nursing homes?

No. Medicare does NOT cover long-term nursing home care, though it will cover up to 100 days of short-term care for problems such as recovering from a fractured hip or a leg ulcer that needs daily dressing changes. Medicare is not designed to pay for the long-term, round-the-clock care needed for AD patients.

Does Medicaid cover nursing homes?

Yes. If a patient's life savings are depleted—then, and only then—will he qualify for Medicaid, the federal program that assists the poor by paying for extended nursing home care. But be forewarned: There may be financial strings attached.

Example: Joseph B. depleted his life savings by paying out-of-pocket to live in a nursing home for two years. Once the money was gone, he qualified for Medicaid, which paid $210,000 for his remaining three years in the facility. Joseph and his wife, Peggy, owned a home, and because Peggy still lived in it, she was allowed to stay there until her death ten years later. When the house sold for $250,000 after Peggy's death, the heirs were shocked to learn they would only get to keep $40,000. Medicaid had placed a lien on the property for the $210,000 of nursing home expenses.

Also, don't kid yourself that you can *hide* Mom's assets by transferring her retirement money to your bank account before applying for Medicaid. Medicaid looks back at the patient's finances for a full five years to see if there have been

---

any large or suspicious movements of money. They also look to see if the home deed was transferred to an heir in an effort to "look poor."

The Take-home Message

There is no free lunch. Nursing homes are expensive and will eat up the retirement savings of most elders in just a few years.

Unless you transfer your parent's money and home more than five years before admission into a nursing home, the government will take their portion of the home equity until the nursing home costs are paid off in full (assuming the patient did not have nursing home insurance or a nest egg large enough to cover the entire stay).

If the home and retirement funds *are* sold or transferred five years before entrance into a nursing home, capital gains and income taxes must be paid on all of the liquidated assets in the year the property was sold or the retirement accounts cashed in. Furthermore, from the day the house deed is transferred, the child will be held liable for property taxes and home owner's insurance, (even though Mom may still be living in the home).

Before such major financial or property transactions are undertaken, an attorney who specializes in elder care issues should be contacted to be sure you fully understand all the monetary and legal ramifications. Your local Alzheimer's Association may be able to assist in selecting a competent elder care attorney.

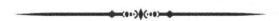

CHAPTER 12

MY EXPERIENCE WITH CAREGIVERS
Dr. Sally Burbank

During my career as a primary care physician, I have witnessed hundreds of families caring for their aging, demented, or disabled loved ones. Some handle it with aplomb and a positive attitude. Others display constant resentment and negativity about the time and energy demanded of them—a real killjoy. The latter seem to thrive on making sure everyone knows how hard it is to be a caregiver and how much they are sacrificing. Their mantra? "I hate it, but what can I do? Woe is me." Even when I suggest alternative options to lessen the burden and allow them to "get a life," they come up with endless excuses and continue to be martyrs. Usually, martyrs provide excellent care, they just complain a lot.

Unfortunately, on several occasions, I have had to intervene when the spouse or children were not providing adequate care. One patient showed up for her doctor's appointment smelling like she hadn't bathed in weeks, and her tattered bathrobe was strewn with last week's mashed potatoes and gravy. Another was losing massive amounts of weight because the pantry and refrigerator were bare, and no one was preparing meals or reminding her to eat. Sometimes prescription medications are taken haphazardly, if at all.

Such neglect is usually not intentional—the kids live far away, have full-time jobs and families of their own, or are still in denial about the severity of Dad's Alzheimer's. Some assume their sibling is looking in on Dad, but in reality, he has reached the point where he can't live alone safely anymore.

Many a son or daughter has told me, "I'm just not the nursing type. I don't want to change diapers or see my father naked." A few, sadly, *willfully* neglect their parent as a spiteful payback. One daughter told me, "Why should I get stuck taking care of him when he was a lousy father? He had an affair, walked out on my mother, and didn't pay child support half of the time. What goes around comes around."

In previous decades, it was assumed that a stay-at-home daughter would take care of her elderly parents. Plus, there were often four or five siblings to help with the workload. Nowadays, most women have fulltime jobs, husbands, children, and even grandchildren to care for, and their time is already stretched thin. There are only so many hours in a day, and members of the "sandwich generation," who are trying to care for their children, grandchildren, and elderly parents, are totally stressed out. Caring for a loved one with AD, or any chronic illness, can be an arduous marathon, but due to the prohibitive cost of nursing homes, most families try to find a way to keep their loved one at home, if at all possible.

~ Caregivers must find a way to get the job done without complete exhaustion or a resentful attitude. ~

The following description of the McClain family is an example of how <u>NOT</u> to do it. (Names and occupations have been changed to protect privacy.)

The Dysfunctional McClain Family

Before he died, Robert McClain made all seven of his children promise they would take care of their mother, Nancy McClain, and NEVER force her to leave her home or enter a nursing home.

The children all dutifully made the deathbed promise with the best of intentions. Five years later, however, when Nancy's Alzheimer's had progressed to moderate severity, the seven siblings weren't prepared for the time-consuming, day-to-day drudgery of taking Mom to countless doctor and dentist appointments, bathing her, making sure her bills were paid, running to the store for prescriptions and groceries, fixing her meals, and making sure she ate nutritious food instead of the sugary junk she preferred. They mowed her yard, cleared her gutters, cleaned her house, did her laundry, and made sure she wasn't left alone too long.

—

Most of the siblings did what they could to help when it was convenient, but they could not be relied upon on a consistent basis.

The oldest son, Greg, thought mowing his mother's stamp-sized yard every other week and changing her light bulbs, air filters, and smoke detector batteries was contributing his fair share of the workload.

Janice, the youngest daughter, only helped when it fit into her jam-packed social calendar. Church meetings, hair appointments, lunch dates with girlfriends, the theater, manicures, her daughter's soccer practices, her son's tennis lessons—all were reasons she cited for not helping more. Yes, when it fit into her schedule, she would visit Mom, do a load of laundry, and even bring a casserole. She might spend ten minutes weeding the flowerbeds, but then she was off to her next scheduled event.

A third sibling, Martin, lived 1,000 miles away and only came for a weekend visit once or twice a year.

The fourth sibling, Kara, was a single mother of three. She worked full time and lived on the opposite side of town—a good forty-minute drive from her mother's house. Kara's contribution was next to nothing because she already felt overwhelmed being a single mother with a full-time job. She felt guilty for not helping more, but she couldn't afford the gas or time to visit her mother more than once a month.

The fifth sibling, Kathy, wasn't on speaking terms with her mother because of a tiff they had three years earlier. Mom apparently made the scathing remark that Kathy's new live-in boyfriend was "a lazy drunk," so Karen refused to help in any way until her mother apologized, which Nancy refused to do, because, with her poor memory, she insisted she never *made* the comment in the first place! (Lord, help me—I should have become a psychiatrist!)

James, the sixth sibling, was an alcoholic, so the family didn't bother asking him for help. "Too unreliable," they all agreed. Even worse? They had to watch Mom's checking account to be sure James hadn't bamboozled his mother into writing him a check, which he promptly wasted on booze.

Because the oldest daughter, Karen, was single, reliable, and lived only ten minutes away, the whole family expected her to do the bulk of the work. "Since you don't have a husband or kids to worry about, it makes sense for you to visit Mom every day before and after work," her sister Janice breezily tossed out.

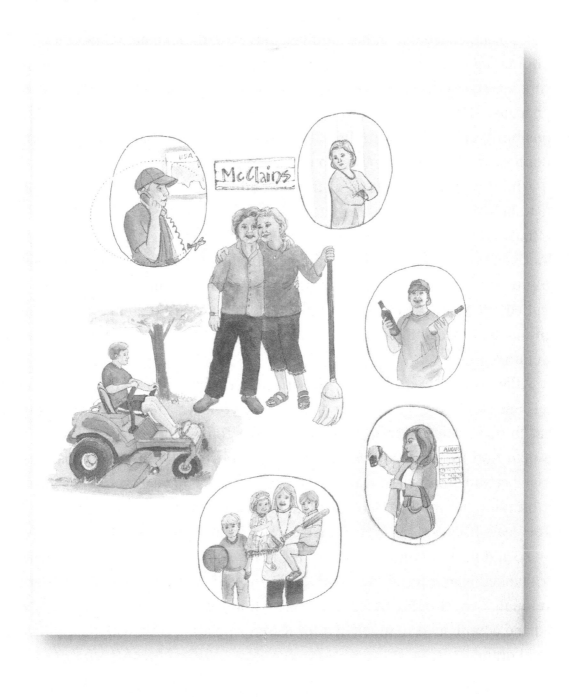

Like the little red hen, Karen did what was expected of her, but she resented how little support she got from her six siblings. Karen never demanded they help, she just wished they would see how overloaded and exhausted she was and volunteer to pitch in more. "Why don't they step up to the plate and do their fair share?" she lamented to me one day. On the rare occasion when she was desperate for back up and called one of her siblings, they would make her feel as though they were doing *her* a favor instead of helping their mother. "I never signed up to be a full-time caregiver," Karen confided, "but somehow the job got dumped on me. Just because I'm single doesn't mean I want to be saddled with the full responsibility and left with no life of my own." She brushed tears from her eyes and confessed, "My life is nothing but drudgery."

And it was! Karen got up every morning at five and drove to her mother's house to help bathe and dress her and walk the dog. Next, she prepared scrambled eggs, toast, and bacon to ensure her mother ate a nutritious breakfast. "Breakfast is Mom's best meal." She then fixed a healthy lunch and left it in the fridge. She made sure her mother took her morning medications, and then dashed off to work. She called her mother mid-morning to check on her, and then again at lunchtime to remind her to eat the sandwich and fruit cocktail on the top shelf of the refrigerator.

After work, she drove back to her mother's house to walk the dog and fix supper. She then spent the evening doing housework and laundry. After getting her mother in bed at nine, Karen drove to her own condo, too exhausted to do much more than flop into bed. She felt sorry for herself but didn't know what to do to improve her situation. All of Karen's sick and vacation days the previous year were spent bringing her mother to medical appointments. Karen hadn't had a vacation in three years because, "Who will take care of Mom while I'm gone?"

To add insult to injury, Nancy McClain was often a demanding patient. She never thanked Karen for all her hard work. Instead, she criticized. "This pot roast is too tough," or, "I don't like beets," or, "I don't want to take a shower." Nancy fretted and complained so much that for Karen, spending time with her mother was a mental drain.

Resentful at the amount of time she had to devote to an ungrateful mother, Karen sometimes snapped at her mother. Several times she even threatened to put her mother in a nursing home if she didn't stop criticizing and complaining. She then would feel guilty because, deep down, she loved her mother and knew it was the Alzheimer's that had changed her mother's personality. Her mother never used to blurt out mean, impulsive remarks before developing the disease.

To make matters worse, when George came every two weeks to mow the yard, Nancy doted on him and lavished him with praise for how much she appreciated all *he* did to help her. Karen seethed. Just because he spent an hour mowing the yard and tightening a leaky faucet, *he* got the praise? Nancy took everything Karen did for granted but waxed eloquent about what a wonderful son George was. "Why doesn't she thank *me* once in a while?" Karen sputtered to me in tears.

The final insult? When Nancy finally died six years later, she had split up the estate equally amongst the seven children. Thus, the alcoholic son who never lifted a finger, (and would likely fritter his money away on booze), and the sister who hadn't spoken to her mother in nine years, obtained exactly the same amount of inheritance as Karen, who had spent a small fortune in gas over the years driving to her mother's house twice a day and escorting her to the doctor.

Even worse? Karen got dumped with the daunting chore of executing the will! More hours of thankless work! Seething with resentment, Karen lashed out at her siblings for not helping more when their mother was alive. Now her relationship with all of her siblings is strained, and after neglecting her friends for six years, she feels alone—and bitter. Talk about The Little Red Hen!!

This is <u>NOT</u> how caretaking is supposed to go!

Some Do's and Don'ts of Family Caregiving

First, never promise you won't put a loved one in a nursing home. No one knows what the future holds, and if the patient becomes violent or impossible to handle, or if the caregiver's health becomes impaired to the point where she doesn't have the energy, time, finances, or health to care for an aging parent or spouse, a nursing home might become necessary. You can only promise, "We will try our best not to let that happen." The family could then joke that Mom might outlive them all!

Second, make a list of every task that needs to be done to care for Mom at home. List everything: driving Mom to her hair and doctor's appointments and weekly church services, balancing the checkbook and paying the bills, cleaning the house, raking the leaves and mowing the yard, buying groceries and picking up prescriptions, bathing, fixing meals, filling her pill caddy each week, getting her to bed and the house locked up.

Third, designate who will do what. If any of the children live out of state, they should agree to send monthly checks to pay for tasks that can be hired out, or to cover the gas and car expenses of those who care for mother. If one child is doing the bulk of the care, they should schedule one day and night a week to get away to go out with friends. Ideally, they also need one full weekend a month to get a break and take care of their own affairs. The other siblings need to write "care for Mom" on their calendars and make it as important as a tennis lesson or hair appointment. If they can't commit to an entire weekend themselves, it is their job to find and pay for a sitter for the time they need to be gone.

Fourth, locate dependable backup, and pay them well. Regular caregivers need to count on every Friday night off, for example, so they can "get a life." If necessary, hire someone to stay with Mom one night a week. Use Mom's retirement accounts to cover the sitter. Remember, paying for the occasional sitter is far less expensive than the $228 per day it costs to live in a nursing home.

Fifth, ask neighbors, grandchildren, nieces, nephews, and church members to assist. Many hands make light work. Not wanting to be a bother, Karen rarely asked anyone for the help she needed, and when she did, she would ask with too little notice. Newsflash: People can't read your mind. Quit being passive. If you need help, ask for it.

Sixth, be specific about what, where, and when you need help. Don't make vague statements such as, "I'm overwhelmed with all the responsibility."

Instead say, "I need someone to change Mom's bed linens and vacuum the house once a month. Could I count on you to sign up for one of these things?"

Seventh, locate a reputable respite care facility nearby. As the caregiver, you might urgently become indisposed or need a week's vacation. Plan ahead.

Eighth, locate an adult daycare or a reliable caregiver to allow you a few scheduled hours each week to run errands. This part-time caregiver could be a friend or church member willing to help. For example, the minister of my parents' small church used to come once a month on a Wednesday at 2:00 p.m. for a "visit." Since my dad would balk at being left with a "babysitter," my mother and the minister always termed it that the minister had "come for a visit." After they conversed for five minutes, my mother would offer cheese and crackers and then say, "Pastor, since you are here to visit with my husband, I'm going to run into town and pick up a few groceries. I'll be right back." She would then drive into town to get her hair done, pick up a few groceries, or stop by the bank and drug store. This allowed her to run errands efficiently while my dad thought the minister was just being sociable. My mother tried to pay the minister for his time, but since my mother was the choir director and pianist, he always refused to take any money.

One time, when Mom's errands lasted over three hours, Dad complained after the minister left. "That guy sure stayed a long time. He wore me out." Mom responded, "He must really like you to have stayed so long. He's told me before how smart he thinks you are." Ego flattered, Dad complained no more about the minister's long visits. Too polite to ask anyone to leave, Dad always played the role of the gracious host, thus allowing Mom to get her errands done.

My mother also had some fabulous retired neighbors who were willing to help in a pinch. If Mom had an appointment, the neighbors would come over for a visit, and Mom would run to her dental cleaning and be back in an hour.

My mother had to *ask* people to help, and she had to ask with enough notice that they could mark it on their calendar. She quickly learned who was reliable. By rounding up multiple people to help, she didn't overtax her volunteers, and by making it a set time each month, the minister had it written on his calendar, and Mom knew which days and times she could schedule her appointments.

Mom also hired the daughter of a close friend to clean her house and change the bed linens twice a month. She paid her generously, so the girl would want to keep coming.

Using these principles, how could the McClain family have handled things better?

First, Martin, the son who lived out-of-state, could have given up one of his two weeks of vacation each year to come stay with his mother. Or, better yet, he could have taken Mom along with *his* family to their Florida beach house, thus allowing Karen to book a one-week vacation of her own. Even if Martin couldn't be there regularly because of the distance, just offering one week a year would have provided Karen a much-needed vacation and mental health break.

Or, Karen and Mom could have joined Martin's family in Florida where Martin could watch Mom some of the time and allow Karen to escape for long walks on the beach each day. Martin and his wife could have insisted on handling all the cooking and laundry, so Karen got a true vacation. Bringing Grandma to the beach house would have had the added benefit of allowing the grandchildren to bond with their "Granny".

Next, the alcoholic son, James, might have been asked to microwave and serve a left-over casserole to his mother one night a week. Many times, even an alcoholic, if he feels needed and included, will rise to the occasion, especially if Karen thanked him profusely each week for his help. It would have been worth a try to include him, though Karen would probably need to lock up Mother's wallet and checkbook before each visit, and not plan anything important on Tuesday nights in case James proved unreliable.

Instead of only mowing the yard for one hour every 2 weeks, George could have come late Saturday afternoon every week to mow the yard, stay through supper, and get his mother to bed. In short, he could have committed to four hours one day a week. This would have allowed Karen an evening to eat out with friends and catch a movie.

Janice, the social butterfly, could have committed to doing her mother's finances during her children's sports practices, and to bringing over a couple casseroles each week. That way, Karen could have had two nights a week she didn't need to prepare meals. Janice could also have committed to cleaning the house twice a month, whenever it fit into her busy schedule, or, she could have hired someone to clean if she didn't have time. Finances, cooking, and housecleaning are time-consuming tasks, but they could have been scheduled into Janice's more unpredictable calendar.

Kara, the single mother, could have brought Mom to church Sunday mornings and then out to a restaurant—paid for by Mom or the wealthier, out-of-state brother, Martin. This would have allowed Kara and her daughters to eat out in a restaurant once a week, and Mom to get out of the house and attend church. It would also have helped Martin to feel he is contributing on a weekly basis to his mother's needs, and it would have given Karen a morning off each week.

Another option would have been for Kara and her daughters to move in with Nancy in exchange for free rent, food, electricity, living expenses, and phone. Once the mother died, it could have been agreed that Kara would inherit the house in exchange for caring for Mom until her death. Or, since Karen did the bulk of the work, the other siblings could have signed over a portion of their share of the estate as a reward for having done ninety percent of the work. They didn't, and now Karen feels resentful and the family is estranged.

Other caregiving options to consider:

Sometimes, a grandchild or reliable college student can live with the AD patient. The grandchild is offered free rent and food in exchange for feeding Granddad breakfast and supper and making sure he takes his meds and gets to bed. It also insures someone is in the house all night. This works in early to mid-AD.

When telling Granddad that a grandchild is staying, do not say, "because you are no longer safe to live alone." He may argue and insist he doesn't need anyone moving in. Instead, tell him the grandchild needs a place to stay because

---

rent is so pricy. My experience with the "greatest generation" is that they are very independent and don't want to be a burden. Thus, make it seem like Grandpa is the one doing the favor. Usually, once the grandchild settles in, things work out fine—so long as the grandchild uses headphones for loud music or video games. In fact, video games are best played in the grandchild's bedroom, if possible. Older people often detest the loud thumps, booms, and explosions emanating from today's rap music and videogames, especially late at night.

If a grandchild goes to live with Grandpa or Grandma, be sure to set up certain ground rules, such as: clean up after yourself, no girlfriends or boyfriends allowed to spend the night, and no making out on the couch when Grandma is up and about. Strangers make Alzheimer's patients uncomfortable, so the plan will only work if the grandchild is considerate, mature, and responsible. If the grandchild is lazy, mouthy, unreliable, or reeks of marijuana, this arrangement will be a disaster! Always make it a "trial run" and put the ground rules in writing.

Here is how one family handled things: Mary, one of eight children, lived with her mother and did all the caretaking. When the mother died, the will split the estate evenly amongst all eight children. This posed a problem because Mary, who had never married, had always lived with her mother. If the estate were split evenly, Mary would suddenly become homeless, as she could not afford to buy out her siblings' share in the house. The other heirs agreed to turn over their share of the house to Mary under the contingency that, when Mary died, she would will it back to her remaining living siblings. They all agreed this seemed fair since Mary had done the bulk of caregiving over many decades. Mary honored her promise, and at her death, the remaining siblings split the estate. Obviously, agreements like this require all members of the family to be selfless and not just looking out for their own immediate financial gain.

Most caregivers perform their tasks selflessly, but it is always nice to feel appreciated by other family members. When my father died, my sister, Ann, flew in from London and stayed a month with my mother who lived in a remote corner of Vermont known as the Northeast Kingdom. Ann, who had been a bank vice president, not only dealt with Dad's Social Security, but also settled his financial affairs, did a thorough housecleaning, hired workers to clean the gutters, had the worn-out carpets pulled up and replaced with beautiful hardwood floors, fixed the aging foundation (so Mom wouldn't have to keep emptying mouse traps, which had always been Dad's job), and helped Mom write thank-you notes to everyone who attended the funeral or sent flowers. On top of that, Ann provided much needed emotional support. Since my siblings and I lived far away, and we all had full-time jobs, we were so grateful to Ann for selflessly giving of her time and talents. I not only wrote her a sincere thank-you note delineating all the things she had done, but I also made sure to mention her considerable sacrifice whenever I spoke to friends and family. My sister didn't make these sacrifices to earn praise, of course, she did them out of love for our mother and to honor our father—who would want his widow taken care of.

Nevertheless, we all appreciate acknowledgement, so if you have a sibling who is doing more than their fair share caring for an ailing parent, be sure to thank them. Send small gifts and be sure to ask what you can do to help.

What Works Best

Many AD patients flatly refuse to leave their homes. The burden they place on their children to take care of all their needs can be overwhelming, especially if the children live more than a few minutes away. Many daughters come to me in tears, overwhelmed and exhausted from trying to care for their parents. They feel they are neglecting their husband and children. "I'm failing everybody," one stressed-out daughter told me. "I spend two hours a day just going to and from my mother's house. I spend all day with her, then rush back to care for my own family. My house is a wreck, and I haven't exercised in months. I've gained twenty pounds, and I'm worn out."

When things reach the point that a caregiver is neglecting her own health and family—or is ready to take a plane to Hawaii and never come back—it is time to make a change! If there are no other available siblings to help, the obvious solution is to have the parent move in with your family. A resistant AD patient will balk, of course, and insist she can stay by herself. When you point out all the things she can no longer do, she will deny it and get furious or accuse you of not loving her. If you try to make Mom understand how worn out you are, she won't. She may act petulant and pouty. She may guilt-trip you in a desperate attempt to avoid moving from her home. Remember, her frontal lobe cannot rationalize normally, so she is clueless about how much time and effort it takes to care for her.

Alzheimer's patients can sometimes be irrational when it comes to long-term planning. They are only capable of thinking about what they want, and they won't grasp the workload required to keep them in their own home. You must consider the needs of not only your loved one, but also your spouse, your children, your job, and your health.

The best arrangement I have seen is when the patient with Alzheimer's has a small space of her own connected to the property of one of the children. It can be inside the home, but it must provide a place for the patient to get away from the hubbub and noise.

When I talk to my elderly patients who have been forced to move in with a child, most of their complaints are about the noise and lack of privacy. In their own home, aside from choosing to watch television or listen to the radio, they had peace and quiet. Elderly patients hate loud music, or the shooting sound of video games, or parents yelling at their kids (or husband!), or kids mouthing off to their parents. Loud arguments between a daughter and son-in-law upset them. A teenager yelling back disrespectfully to his mother is distressing. Remember, the patient mirrors the emotions of the home.

Provide as much privacy as possible. AD patients want to watch their favorite TV programs, so they should have a television in their bedroom. Load up the fridge and pantry with their favorite healthy foods and allow them to decorate their bedroom and bathroom as they see fit. Provide a comfortable chair or recliner in their bedroom in front of the TV. Try to avoid arguments and shouting within Mom's hearing.

Don't sell Mom's house the minute you move her into your home. The move may turn into a disaster. Inform Mom the move into your home is a trial run for three months to see how it goes. Tell her you can no longer drive across town every day without neglecting your own family, and you love her too much to see her not properly cared for. Don't argue with her. If she insists she doesn't want to move, say, "I understand, Mom, but this is the way it has to be." When she brings up that she wants to go home, stay calm and say things like, "I know you do, Mom. You have the prettiest roses." In short, validate her feelings but then immediately change the subject.

Be sure you bring her bed, pillow, bedspread, favorite chair, TV, and favorite photos. The goal is to make Mom's bedroom seem familiar and as much like her own home as possible.

Sometimes you can help Mom feel more a part of the family by asking her to help with folding towels, peeling potatoes, or watering flowers. Most parents enjoy feeling needed and useful, and they will feel like a welcomed part of the family, and less like a burden, if you include them.

If your home isn't big enough to provide a private living space for Mom, discuss building a small addition to your home that includes a bedroom with a private bath and a small living room. If the addition allows a separate outside entrance from the rest of the family, the space can later be rented out to offset some of the building costs. Be sure the space is built on the main level without the need for stairs.

Since the addition is specifically being built to house your mother, Mom's retirement money or Social Security could be used to build it. Remember, one year in a nursing home costs $80,000, so if a small efficiency apartment could be built for $40,000 dollars or so, it is still less than half a year in the nursing home. Some families turn an unfinished basement, recreation room, or garage space into separate living quarters. Stairs are often a problem with this plan since recreation rooms and basements often require navigating a flight of stairs. Early on, the patient can usually navigate stairs, but as the disease progresses, stairs become dangerous. AD patients lose spatial judgment and balance, and falls are common. Perhaps for the final year or so of a parent's life, the caregivers could sleep in the basement bedroom and let Mom sleep in the main level bedroom. Or, a simple foldout couch could be placed in a first-floor den or study and function as Mom's bedroom.

I have seen siblings balk at the idea of Mom cashing in $40,000 of retirement money to build an addition onto one of the children's homes. In the mind of the other siblings, one sister is getting a "free" $40,000 home improvement, which means there will be that much less in the estate to split up when Mom dies. My advice is to tell the complaining siblings that if they want to move Mom into their home and volunteer to be responsible for feeding, bathing, driving, and caring for her day in and day out, 24/7, then by all means, put the addition onto *their* home instead—but with the "free" addition comes the day-to-day responsibility of caring for Mom until she dies. Usually, the complaining siblings shut up when faced with this choice. It also helps to remind the quibbling siblings that if Mom went into a nursing home instead of your house, her retirement savings and potentially the entire equity of her home would be used up, and there would be *nothing* left in the estate to split.

In many families, there is a "Monday morning quarterback" who loves to criticize and tell you what you are doing wrong in your caregiving of Mother. This know-it-all often won't lift a finger to help—he or she just likes to inform you of what *you* should be doing differently. Often this person will spend thirty minutes with Mom once a week and think you are exaggerating about how bad Mom has gotten, mainly because Mom always looks well-fed and bathed—thanks to you! Know-it-alls can be more irksome than Mom's repetitive questions!

Unfortunately, Mom will try to convince this less involved family member—let's call him Paul—that she is perfectly fine on her own and doesn't need any help, and certainly doesn't need to move in with you. Mom will insist you are forcing her out of her home against her will.

Paul doesn't grasp that Mom can no longer drive to the grocery store, take her meds properly, change out of her bathrobe, or remember to shower if you aren't there every day to oversee things. When he comes for a visit, he sees a vacuumed house and Mom dressed in clean clothes. He opens the door to a full pantry and is convinced you are exaggerating the severity of Mom's condition.

What he *doesn't* see is how much time you spend making all this happen! He doesn't see how much you neglect your own family and health by driving across town to cater to Mom's needs on a daily basis. Mom likely won't acknowledge all you do for her because she doesn't remember everything you do— she has Alzheimer's! Your brother may minimize everything you do because he isn't ready to accept Mom's downward trajectory, or, he doesn't want to share the blame in forcing his mother out of her home.

Obviously, you *should* carefully consider the advice offered by your siblings. Don't take every suggestion as a personal attack or criticism. Defensiveness and family squabbles will not help your mother! Keep in mind your siblings may see things you don't, so be open to their practical suggestions. They care about Mother too, even if they cannot share the responsibilities equally.

Unrelenting criticism by other family members only adds to your stress. Sometimes you have to take the high road and do the right thing, even if you get criticized for it. Remember: if your siblings aren't intimately participating in Mom's care, they cannot see the depth of her needs. Perhaps you should invite the family critic to spend one week with Mother, so he can better witness her declining abilities.

In summary, caregivers need to elicit help from others to avoid burnout. Don't rely on people volunteering on their own. When asked, many are willing to help, so ask for it!

CHAPTER 13

———◆◆◆———

DAY-TO-DAY MANAGEMENT
Sue Bell

Organization and Efficiency

Becoming organized gives you a sense of control in situations where you feel like you have none.

Many retired people have the luxury of a somewhat slower, more relaxed pace. The kids are finally grown and out of the house, and there is no longer a job requiring a strict schedule and rush hour traffic. When a loved one gets diagnosed with AD, however, the caregiver quickly discovers it is time to get organized and time-efficient.

There are many reasons for this. Preparing meals for and feeding a patient with AD takes more time, as does bathing and dressing. AD patients tend to walk slower, fall more often, or need assistance with things they used to do independently. While eating, they may spill their milk, stain their clothes, or pour their beverage onto their plate, ruining their meal. This means preparing another plate of food, cleaning the floor, and more dirty laundry.

Since AD patients are notorious for wandering off or losing (or hiding) things, you will squander time finding your patient or the items they squirrel away in the most unpredictable locations.

After Ray was diagnosed with AD, I spent a lot of time looking for misplaced items. I scrambled to get supper on the table while watching my husband to make sure he hadn't roamed off—again. Even though I was retired, I didn't have enough time to get everything done. I suffered from a perpetual lack of sleep and exhaustion. It reminded me of when I had three children at home under the age of

———

six. I had to become proactive in my organization and time management. Over the years, I discovered many timesaving ideas. So, what helped most?

Make a Schedule

A schedule lets you feel in control of all that must be done. Be sure to include time for yourself during the day to counteract the feeling that your life is controlled by AD. "Me" time should be something you love doing, such as reading, playing a musical instrument, painting, gardening, or watching a favorite TV show.

~ Schedule "me" time and make it a priority. Even if it is only thirty minutes, you need something to look forward to each day. ~

It is not selfish to need time for yourself, so don't swallow up this cherished time with dirty laundry. Keeping a schedule helped me know I could complete all the "have to" chores and still get my precious hour of reading.

Sue's Typical Daily Schedule:

6:00 a.m.	Get up. Get Ray showered, shaved, and dressed for the day.
7:00 a.m.	Have a cup of coffee together on the porch. Read the paper while Ray watches the birds and enjoys the flowers. Take Ray and the dog for a walk.
8:00 a.m.	Eat breakfast and clean up the kitchen. Start a load of wash.
9:00 a.m.	Put clothes in the dryer. Feed the birds, deadhead flowers. Do light housekeeping with Ray: vacuuming, dusting, emptying the dishwasher, and folding laundry.
11:00 a.m.	Read a book. I considered this my sacred time, and I tried to make sure reading was in my daily schedule. Ray would nap or explore

	the "mystery boxes" filled with interesting items for him to investigate while I read.
12:00 p.m.	Make sack lunches and walk to the park to eat with Ray.
1:00 p.m.	Go for a joy ride on back roads, visit a friend, or run errands in town. Stop for ice cream.
3:00 p.m.	Come home. Work a simple jigsaw puzzle together or look at picture books. Play with the dog or let Ray play golf in the hallway using a golf ball, a putter, and a plastic cup turned on its side.
6:00 p.m.	Eat supper and load dishwasher. Sit on the porch with Ray and enjoy the evening.
7:00 p.m.	Watch Ray's favorite television channel (the one with cowboy movies). Make phone calls, pay the bills, or catch up on Facebook while he watches his program.
9:30 p.m.	Prepare for bed.
10:00 p.m.	Lights out.

It may sound simple, but following this schedule gave me a feeling of control. Since my doctor had talked with me about the importance of daily exercise, I made my daily walk a high priority. Even if your patient cannot be left alone, you can still incorporate exercise into your routine by purchasing a used exercise bicycle or working out to DVDs. You can also put on some lively music and make up dance steps with the patient. Why? Exercise relieves stress and helps prevent depression by raising endorphin levels.

Organization

- Keep everything in a specific place and always put it back after use.
- Keep updated lists of all needed items, including groceries, on the refrigerator.
- Keep an updated list of errands that need to be done so you can consolidate your trips. It is difficult to leave home during the later stages, so combining errands is critical.
- Pay bills electronically by automatic withdrawal or on the computer.
- Place the mail in a specific place out of sight of the patient.

Meal Preparation

- Plan meals ahead to minimize trips to the grocery store. Shop from a list.
- Keep items on hand to prepare quick meals at any time—pasta and sauce, macaroni and cheese dinners, peanut butter and jelly, canned soups, frozen lasagna, TV dinners, frozen meatloaf.
- When you cook, make double portions and freeze what you don't need now for later. Store left-overs in single-meal containers and label with the current date.
- Use crockpots for easy meal preparation and make enough for several meals or enough to freeze.
- Have plenty of finger foods and grab-and-go snacks available. Try to include healthy, nutritious snacks, such as string cheese, fruits and veggies, protein bars, nuts, whole-grain crackers with hummus, yogurt, or peanut butter and crackers.
- Use a hand towel for a placemat. This keeps spilled food from damaging the furniture or dripping onto the floor. Towels are easy to wash. Use a bath towel in the patient's lap to protect clothing.

- Use large adult-sized bibs during feeding. You can also use hand towels as bibs. If the patient balks that bibs are for babies, wear one yourself.

- Serve soup in a mug, not a bowl, to prevent dribbling.

Visitors

- Allow the patient to have visitors. It pleases her, even if she doesn't recognize the visitor anymore.

- Be sure to let visitors know in private that the patient may not recognize them or know their name. Let the patient serve cookies and lemonade to the guests, if they are still able. Let Mom feel like the hostess.

- Keep old photos from the patient's childhood on the coffee table to serve as conversation starters with guests. Hang photos of vacation spots or favorite scenic vistas on the wall.

- Introduce visitors at the onset of the visit and remind the patient how she knows the guest. This allows the patient to save face and will keep the guest from asking, "Do you remember who I am?" By saying something like, "Richard Jones from the church choir has come to visit us," you can prevent your loved one from feeling humiliated when she doesn't remember his name or how she knows him.

Household Duties

- Before Alzheimer's, your loved one likely performed many household chores. Now that he is unable to do those tasks without supervision, who will keep up the car maintenance (oil and filter changes, tune-ups, winter tires) and home maintenance (changing air filters and ceiling light bulbs, cleaning the gutters, shoveling snow, mowing the grass, or trimming the hedges)? You will either need to learn how to do these tasks yourself or locate family or friends or hired workers to take over the task. Word of mouth is often the best way to find a reliable handyman.

- Keep a list of handymen with names and phone numbers readily available.
- Sally's mother jokingly said she most missed her husband when the mousetraps needed emptying and when the electricity went off in the dead of winter in northern Vermont. Since she didn't know how to run a gas generator, her mother would bundle up in four layers of clothing, including a bulky ski parka, and wait for the electricity to be restored. (Gas generators had always been her father's domain.)

Laundry

- Keep changes of clothes readily accessible. Once, after getting Ray ready to go out, he walked into the kitchen, picked up a cup of coffee, and spilled it all over his shirt. New clothes needed!
- Spray clothes for stains immediately. Carry stain sticks in your purse in case the spill occurs in a restaurant.
- Warning: Laundry can quickly become overwhelming. Do it daily to keep odors from growing.

Reduce the Risk of Falls

- Install ramps, handrails, and grab bars where needed.
- In the bathroom, provide shower chairs with arms, handheld showerheads, and raised toilet seats. Have no-slip grips on the bottom of the tub and grab bars if needed to prevent falls.
- Get rid of all throw or scatter rugs. They are a major cause for falls.

~ All stairs must have sturdy railings! No excuses. Get it done! ~

Bedtime

- One lady would lead her husband to bed every night by walking backward, holding both of his hands as he walked forward down the hall. She would sing a lullaby while they walked, and they would shake hands once they reached the bedroom. This would make him laugh. She was able to coax him to the bedroom at night because of this simple routine.

- Divide preparing for bedtime into simple steps: Walk to bathroom. Brush teeth. Wash face. Empty bladder. Put on two pairs of clean pull-ups. Get into pajamas, and so on.

- Don't wait too long to get started with the bedtime routine. Overtired patients become cranky and uncooperative.

- Do NOT share tomorrow's schedule with patients at bedtime. Caregivers may think informing patients ahead of time about tomorrow's agenda will make them more cooperative in the morning. Wrong! AD patients often obsess about upcoming appointments and have trouble falling asleep. They may get confused and get up at 3:00 a.m., convinced it is time to get dressed and eat breakfast so they won't be late for their doctor's appointment or church. The caregiver will then be awakened and have great difficulty convincing the patient church isn't for another seven hours. The patient will continue to worry about missing the appointment or church service and may not be able to fall back asleep—until 9:00 a.m.—when the caregiver needs the patient to get up.

~ Many AD patients have no sense of time, and advanced notice about future plans only makes them fret and ruminate. The patient does not need to know tomorrow's plans—only the caregiver. ~

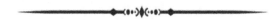

CHAPTER 14

FOOD, GLORIOUS FOOD!
Sue Bell and Dr. Sally Burbank

Do I make my loved one eat healthy food, or do I let him eat what he wants? Like an obstinate child, an AD patient can be a picky eater. You need to choose which battles to fight because you can't make a patient eat, and an addled AD patient may overturn his entire dinner plate if you push him too hard to eat Brussels sprouts. Even worse, he may throw his unwanted zucchini in your face—or toss it to the dog.

Unfortunately, many AD patients only want junk food or sweets. Raw veggies and tofu? Not so much! Others insist on one or two specific items, such as macaroni and cheese or canned peaches, and then refuse to eat the other items you prepared.

I allowed Ray to eat what he wanted. Hamburgers, French fries, chocolate, breakfast cereal, and ice cream were allowed on his diet. My philosophy: Why not let him have a little comfort and happiness, if that's what he wants? Food remained one of his few remaining pleasures. By letting him eat what he wanted, he remained calm and non-aggressive, and it avoided needless arguments and power struggles. Alzheimer's is a terminal disease. Sure, eating super healthy might have prolonged his life a couple of months, but for what? So he could endure more months of end-stage Alzheimer's? I chose to keep him happy, even if it meant he died a few months sooner than he would have had I insisted on only super-healthy foods. Not everyone will agree with my decision, of course, but that's the path I chose.

Ray loved mealtime and seemed to engage with me while eating. As the disease progressed, I would sometimes have to feed him a bite or two to get him started. I would then transfer the spoon to his hand and guide his hand toward the

---

plate and then back to his mouth. Once I reminded him how to eat, he would continue on his own. The last few weeks of his life, I had to partially feed him by guiding his spoon from his plate to his mouth on every bite, but he was able to eat until the day he died.

Caregivers often have strong opinions about food, but here are a few guiding principles we recommend:

Guiding Food Principles

• Eat with the patient at a table. It makes mealtime more enjoyable and encourages the patient to eat more. Avoid eating in front of the television, as patients are easily distracted and will eat less if they are engrossed in a program. Choking is also reduced if the patient is sitting up fully in a chair when eating.

• Don't give patients hard candy, suckers, Jell-O, or other choking hazards. Surprisingly, chewing gum is not usually a problem if their teeth are good and they don't wear dentures. Most patients will chew sugar-free gum for hours which helps clean their teeth.

• While some patients must strictly control their intake of sweets because of diabetes, the majority of patients can be allowed a little freedom in the area of food choice. Comfort foods are one of the simple pleasures that Alzheimer's cannot rob from a patient, and a desired treat can improve the patient's mood. Allow your loved one to enjoy their favorite foods within the scope of an overall balanced diet.

• Explaining the health benefits of broccoli will get you nowhere. It is better for the patient to eat scrambled eggs and toast every day for a month than to eat nothing, (because he doesn't like what you fixed), and lose ten pounds. Sneak in healthy foods by tucking extra powdered milk into a milkshake or putting veggies into a lasagna to increase the nutritional value. Add pureed veggies to tomato soup and serve the soup in a mug.

• As the disease progresses, Alzheimer patients lose the ability to recognize hunger cues. Either that, or they lack the verbal ability to ask you to prepare them something to eat. Thus, to encourage them to eat, leave healthy snacks such as peanut butter crackers, cut-up grapes, Chex mix, fruit cocktail or cut up peaches or pears next to their favorite chair. If food is in plain sight, they might eat it.

• Have the patient drink one nutrient-rich shake every day such as Boost Plus or Ensure Plus. Diabetics may prefer Glucerna which is low in sugar.

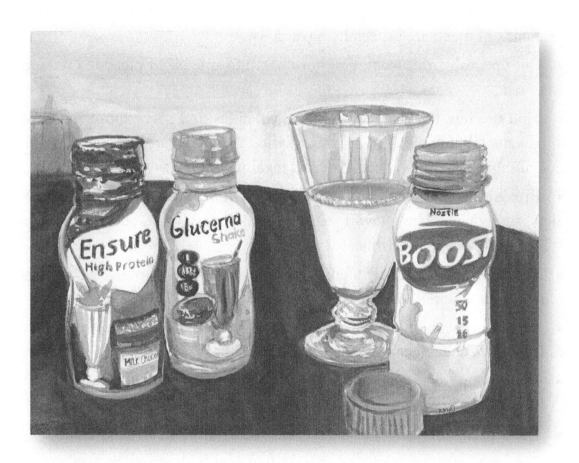

• If the patient is losing weight, serve Boost Plus with each meal instead of a calorie-free or nutrient-poor beverage such as water, coffee, soda, or tea. Serve it cold and in a glass, not straight from the can so it will seem like a part of the meal and not a supplement. Boost Plus provides a whopping 360 calories per can and comes in chocolate, strawberry, and vanilla. Ensure Plus has additional flavors, so if the patient doesn't like one, try another. You can also make your own smoothies with protein powder, frozen fruits, and yogurt. Eggnog and boiled custard are also nutrient-rich. The Plus version of Boost or Ensure provides four additional grams of protein and 140 additional calories over the plain Boost and Ensure.

- In late-stage AD, choking becomes a risk, as patients forget to chew thoroughly and even how to swallow. Certain foods, such as whole grapes, large chunks of pineapple or fresh fruit, hot dogs, dry hard rolls or bread, popcorn, and large chunks of meat, are especially hazardous.

- Cut up fresh fruit, meat, and hot dogs into bite-sized pieces to reduce the choking risk.

- Find the few healthy foods the patient likes and serve those foods often. Most patients fall into a dull monotony of what they will eat. Perhaps the best way to look at this new reality is that it makes meal planning easy.

- Breakfast is often their best meal, so make it healthy. Serve scrambled eggs, omelets, smoothies, Greek yogurt with granola, cheesy toast, cottage cheese with fruit, ham and biscuits, or oatmeal with fruit.

- Purchase large-handled utensils from Amazon. A "spork"—combination fork and spoon—works well for many.

- Serve beverages in plastic cups to avoid shattered glass splaying across the room if the patient accidentally knocks one over.

- Fill drinking cups only half full to avoid spills. You can always refill the cup.

- Use a plastic tablecloth or hand towel for a placemat for easy clean up.

- Buy matching large bibs or smocks that you both wear for meals to avoid ruining clothes. If you wear one too, the patient won't feel ashamed or singled out.

- Use plastic plates with divided sections (picnic plates) so the patient has a lip to push against. This will prevent food from being pushed off the plate onto the table.

- Serve soup in a mug, not a bowl. Manual dexterity declines over time, and mugs allow the patient to drink the broth, thus preventing soiling their clothes.

- Serve finger foods—they are less messy and frustrating. Try fish sticks, French fries, whole green beans, toast, boiled eggs, chicken fingers, small slices of pizza, cooked baby carrots, and sandwiches cut into four squares.

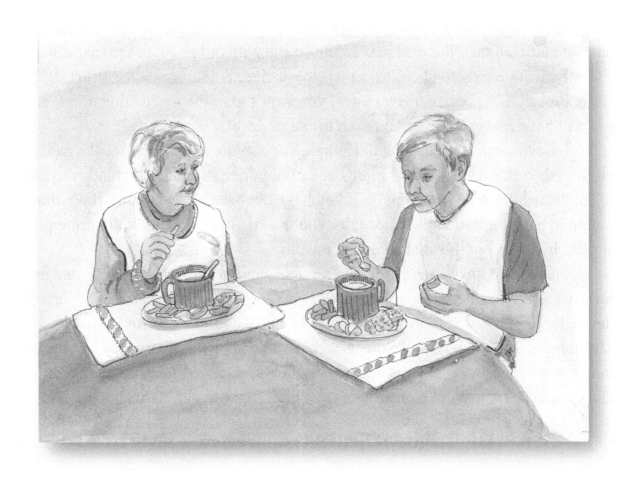

What if your patient is diabetic and stubbornly refuses to eat a healthy diet?

In these patients, be careful with any diabetes medications that can bottom out their sugars, such as glyburide, glipizide, or glimepiride. If a patient takes one of these medications before eating and then eats only two bites, his blood sugar can bottom out and become dangerously low. I advise caregivers to have the patient eat first and *then* take the medication only if the patient has eaten the majority of his carbohydrate-rich foods, (i.e. cereal, toast, rice, potato, pasta, or fruit). With this approach, if he only eats two bites, you won't give the medication at all, and you will have prevented bottoming out his sugar level.

I use the same approach with Humalog or Novolog insulin. Have the patient eat first, then size up how many grams of carbohydrate the patient actually ate and adjust the insulin dose accordingly. If you have not been educated in carbohydrate counting, have the patient's doctor refer you to a dietitian to go over the principles of carbohydrate counting and adjusting insulin.

Thankfully, the American Diabetes Association now says elderly patients need not strive for the same stringent sugar control as younger patients. In fact, a Hemoglobin A1C of less than 9 is now deemed good enough for patients with Alzheimer's. Why? Too many patients were ending up in the emergency room with dangerously low sugars when caregivers and doctors aimed for normal sugars. In short, a low sugar is more dangerous than a high sugar in elderly diabetics.

~ Even in late-stage AD, patients appreciate a tasty treat! ~

• Nancy N. was in a nursing home that did not allow her to have sweets, so her family occasionally snuck in her favorite dessert. She no longer recognized her husband or daughter, but her face lit up when she was offered a homemade chocolate chip cookie.

• Sarah S. regrets she didn't fix hot dogs for her husband more often. They were his favorite food, but she didn't serve them because she felt they were unhealthy. After he passed, she felt guilty for not serving him the treat he loved. In the long run, would it have mattered if he died a month or two sooner because he had eaten a hot dog every couple of weeks?

- Dorothy W. coaxed her thin husband into drinking a can of Boost Plus at lunchtime every day by bribing him. Her husband loved root beer, but she made him "earn" it first by drinking a full can of Boost Plus. He would sputter, but he always complied because he looked forward to sipping on his beloved can of root beer all afternoon. Similar bribes can be tried using your patient's favorite treat.

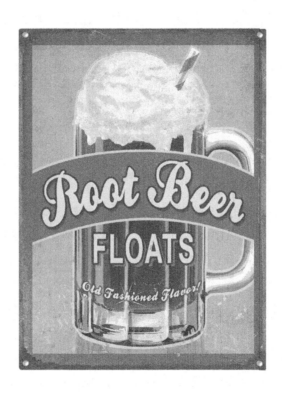

CHAPTER 15

●‹‹›❖‹‹›●

PERSONAL HYGIENE
Sue Bell

When caring for your patient, you may think you need the training of a nurse, but thankfully, all the skills you need can be easily learned. While personal care can be a challenge, appearance and hygiene matter—even if the patient is no longer capable of taking care of those needs himself. Appearance impacts other people's perceptions of your loved one—and you. You can honor your loved one by taking the time to help him look presentable, even if he no longer seems to care. Here are some suggestions:

Bathing

Bathing an Alzheimer's patient can be frustrating. As with all tasks, common sense and patience go a long way.

First, establish a bathing routine. In the early stages, most patients will be able to take care of bathing without much assistance. They may just need reminders and gentle prodding to shower. As the disease progresses, however, your loved one will need an increasing level of supervision. By the late stage, some patients are bed-bound and will rely on you completely for sponge baths.

How often should a memory-challenged elderly patient bathe or shower? Skin becomes dry with age, and bathing too frequently is actually harmful, as it causes itching and flakiness. Thus, two or three times a week is generally sufficient, especially if the person is inactive and doesn't sweat much. When the hair looks greasy or flat, it is a sign it needs washing.

There are four options when assisting your patient with bathing: a regular standing shower, a bath (sitting in the tub), a shower while sitting in a shower chair, or a sponge bath. Sponge baths can be used between showers or tub baths to save time. The hands, face, underarms, and groin areas should be washed daily with a warm washcloth. Always wipe from front to back in the groin area to prevent urinary tract infections in women.

Gather up every needed item—shampoo, liquid soap, razors, moisturizing lotions, deodorant, washcloths, and towels—ahead of time, and store them in a plastic caddy. As with a baby or toddler, never leave your patient alone in the tub or shower while you dash off to find a forgotten item. In the one minute you are gone, the patient can become anxious and attempt to leave the shower or tub. Falls and

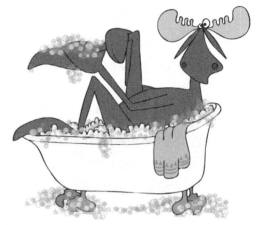

drowning can occur in the short time you are gone. Even though you tell her, "I'll be right back," or, "Stay right here," she won't *remember* when you are out of sight, and she may attempt to come find you.

If the bathroom is chilly, first warm up the room with an electric heater until it is toasty warm. Patients chill easily and will resist removing their clothes if the room is too cold. Better a little too warm than too cold. Towels warmed in the dryer make the experience pleasant for patients.

Baby shampoo works best in case the shampoo gets in her eyes. It is also gentle and hypoallergenic.

AD patients sometimes become afraid of forcefully running water. If the patient seems fearful, fill up the tub *before* you bring her into the bathroom. Also, some patients are easily startled by sudden loud noises, so turn the water on and off slowly to avoid frightening her.

One patient became frightened of the forceful pressure of the water faucet. She pulled back with wide eyes and told the nurse, "I can't swim!"

Likewise, strong water pressure from a forceful showerhead or tub faucet can be painful on sensitive, elderly skin. If you notice red streaks, or if she resists bathing, the shower pressure may be too strong. Be careful with temperature, as well—too hot or too cold and the patient may fight you. Test the temperature with your elbow. Patients prefer the water temperature warm but not hot.

Warn your patient what you are about to do. For example, "I am now going to wash your back with this washcloth." Hold up the washcloth so she can see it. Speak in a pleasant calm tone and then make conversation to distract your patient. Finish as quickly as possible, as the attention span of an AD patient is short.

Avoid spraying water on the patient's face. If the patient is still able to assist you, demonstrate how to stroke and gently clean the face with a warm washcloth.

Some patients are modest and will shy away from someone seeing their naked body. She has been accustomed to privacy while bathing her entire adult life. To make the patient more comfortable, keep the shower curtain partially pulled to allow as much privacy as possible.

If your patient is taking a tub bath or is sitting in a shower chair, you can place a small hand towel over her private areas. Allow your patient to help as much as possible—this helps her retain her dignity. Try giving her a warm, wet washcloth and ask her to wash her arms as you clean other areas. You may have to demonstrate how to do this. If you keep her distracted with her own washcloth, she will be less likely to fight you as you clean her groin and breasts.

While you wash her legs, neck and face, keep her breasts and groin area covered with a bath towel to preserve her privacy if she is modest. Leave the towel covering the groin in place while you wash the breasts. If she resists you removing the towel from her breasts or privates, leave the towel on and clean with a washcloth underneath the towel. This allows you to clean without making her feel exposed. Ask the patient to hold the bath towel so her hands are occupied. This keeps her from pushing your hand away.

For some patients, you can distract them from their discomfort with a cheery song. Try singing, "This is the way we wash our arms, wash our arms, wash our arms. This is the way we wash our arms so early in the morning." This is a familiar tune, and the patient may sing along. You can then sing, "This is the way we wash our chest," and so on until the body is clean. By singing the same song at every bath, it can become a ritual.

As the disease progresses, a bed bath or sponge bath may be all you can do. Always use the soft side of a washcloth and a gentle touch to avoid bruising or breaking the skin, which can lead to infection. Several companies offer disposable washcloths that can be used without water, making even the most challenging baths easier.

Dry shampoo can be used to avoid startling the patient with water around her face.

Whatever method you choose to bathe your patient, do it with a smile on your face. Avoid acting put out with the patient if she resists you. Instead, try distraction and getting her involved by holding the towel or washcloth.

Helpful hygiene items to consider purchasing include shower chairs with arms, (which are safer than cheap plastic lawn chairs that are prone to tipping over), bath benches, handrails, special basins, hair trays, no-slip bath mats, raised commode seats, and cushioned commode seats if the patient is thin. Hand-held shower nozzles are a must if the patient is sitting in a chair or if you are assisting with the shower. They can be installed cheaply, and they prevent the patient from getting water in her face.

If possible, have patients empty their bladder and bowels in the toilet before showering, even if they insist they don't need to go. Warm water can trigger patients to have an accident in the shower or tub. If this happens, don't embarrass or shame them by fussing—they can't control their bodily functions anymore, and they don't do it on purpose. Stay calm and act as though it's no big deal. If you act upset, it will make them more resistant to bathing in the future.

Dental Care

Ideally, the patient's teeth should be brushed twice each day and flossed daily, but as the disease advances, this becomes harder and harder to accomplish. In the early and middle stages, you might only need to remind your loved one to brush. In the middle stage, you will have to apply the toothpaste to the brush and show him how to brush by demonstrating on your own teeth. Patients who have always used an electric toothbrush may continue to accept it, but others may become afraid of the noise and motion.

When patients reach the moderate to severe stage, you will have to brush their teeth for them. That's when the problems start. Most patients bite the toothbrush thinking it is food or something to chew on. The only solution I found was letting Ray bite on the hard, plastic side of a toothbrush turned sideways on one side of his mouth while I brushed the other side with a second toothbrush. I then changed which side he chewed on while I brushed the opposite side.

In the later stages, the patient may not grasp the concept of spitting out the toothpaste, even if you demonstrate how to spit. Luckily, toothpaste is not toxic if swallowed, but to reduce the risk of aspiration, you may need to abandon toothpaste altogether and go to Plan B: Dip the toothbrush in mouthwash and just brush with that, using a second toothbrush for the patient to bite on. You may have to dip the brush in mouthwash multiple times to get both sides of their mouth clean.

Flossing became nearly impossible after the early stage, so I eventually quit trying and had to settle for gently brushing Ray's gums with a soft toothbrush.

If your patient has dentures, be sure to remove and clean them. Use a soft cloth adhered to a toothbrush to clean their gums. Never stick your fingers in their mouth, or you will likely be bitten—a lesson I learned the hard way!

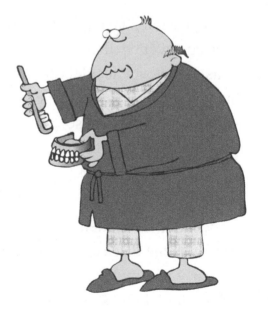

Patients often enjoy chewing sugarless gum, which freshens the breath and removes food particles from the teeth.

One patient, Alene P., would grimace when eating or when someone brushed her teeth. The dentist could find no obvious problem, although he admitted the exam was less than ideal because she wouldn't cooperate when he tried to examine her or perform X-rays. She clamped her jaw closed and refused to open up. Even with attempts to pry her mouth open, the dentist couldn't see well enough to discover the problem. She was sent home with no definitive cause found. Eventually, a rotten tooth fell out of her mouth. It was missed at her appointment because she wouldn't cooperate with the dental exam. Thus, it is best to get a thorough exam with X-rays when the patient is still in the early stages. Get any needed dental work done while the patient is still cooperative.

Shaving

In the early and middle stages, you may just have to remind your loved one to shave, but eventually, supervision and assistance will be necessary. When your patient begins cutting his face on a regular basis, it is time to take over. If your loved one has always used an electric razor, he may continue to do so, or he may let you use the electric razor.

During the early and middle stages of his disease, Ray would not allow me to use an electric razor, as he seemed to fear the noise. Our doctor suggested I do the shaving with a regular razor but have him hold an electric razor that was not turned on—so he wouldn't grab my hand. Eventually, in the very late stage, he did allow me to use an electric razor, which was much quicker.

Moral of the story: If something doesn't work the first time, don't give up. It may work later on.

One time, Ray would not allow me to shave him. I was in a hurry because we had an appointment. The more impatient and insistent I became, the more he resisted, so I stopped altogether. Instead, I distracted him by pointing out his reflection in the mirror. I made small talk about the handsome guy staring back at us. I smiled, patted his shoulder, and distracted him for several minutes. I then began to ask him questions about the man in the mirror—what color his eyes were, how much hair he had, etc. As Ray concentrated on the reflection, which he did not recognize as his own, I was able to shave him.

Distraction remains a caregiver's best ally. Why? Because in the later stages, the patient seems capable of only focusing on one thing at a time.

By getting Ray to focus on how much hair the man in the mirror had, I was able to get him shaved. If shaving becomes too much of a headache, let the patient grow a beard. Trim the beard using sharp, blunt-tipped scissors when the patient is asleep on his back.

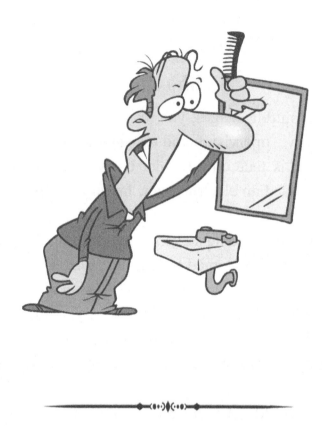

CHAPTER 16

DRESS FOR SUCCESS
Sue Bell

Best Clothing Choices

Clothing should be loose and comfortable. In the late stage, many patients sit all day, so pants that are too fitted can feel constricting. Since buttoning a shirt or tying a shoelace can be difficult, patients become frustrated and quit trying to dress themselves. The solution? Buy clothes that make dressing easy.

Safety, comfort, and ease are king when choosing clothing. Items must be easy to put on: elastic waists, Velcro straps, pullover tops. Loungewear that is comfortable and soft works well. Loose pullover tops and a light cardigan or jacket that opens all the way down the front are simple to get on and off. Bright colors seem to appeal to many AD patients.

~ Elastic waistband pants in a size larger than normal are easier to pull down quickly in the bathroom and can help minimize accidents. ~

Purchase loose pants with belt loops, but instead of wearing a belt, tie a shoelace between the two loops on the back of the pants to keep the pants up. When they need to undress, untie the lace and let the pants drop to the floor without having to struggle to undo buttons or snaps. This technique also works great for changing adult diapers or underwear quickly.

Walking around in stocking feet can cause falls, often resulting in broken bones. Purchase non-slip grip socks. These may be worn without shoes. Tube socks are easy to pull on when shoes are worn. Shoelaces are problematic—the patient cannot tie his own shoes, and he can trip over untied laces. Slip-on shoes or shoes

---

with Velcro closures are a good choice. If local stores don't have them, buy them on-line.

As the disease progresses and the patient loses weight, they often complain of being cold. Jogging suits can solve this problem. One strong-minded Alzheimer's patient had shopped only in high-end department stores her entire life. Each and every day, she dressed in her "Sunday best" dresses. When she moved to a nursing home, her daughter purchased several sets of colorful velveteen jogging suits at Wal-Mart and brought them to her mother. Her mother couldn't believe how soft and comfortable they were. "I don't know where these have been all my life," she commented. After that, she wouldn't wear anything else.

Incontinence

As the disease progresses, do not rely on the patient's ability to tell you when she needs to go to the bathroom. If you do, you will face piles of urine-soaked clothes, mounting frustration, and a humiliated patient. Never shame the patient for having an accident—she can't help it.

If the patient begins to have accidents, it is time to employ a timed voiding approach. Timed voiding means every two hours the patient goes to the bathroom whether she feels like it or not. Some caregivers set a timer to go off every two hours and matter-of-factly inform the patient it is time to go to the bathroom. Patients will frequently balk and insist, "I don't need to go." When this happens—and it will—calmly explain that Alzheimer's patients lose the ability to tell when they need to go, so they need to at least try every two hours. If this fails—and it will—say, "I know you don't feel like you need to go, but there's no harm in trying. Besides, it's good for us to get up and stretch our legs." Then distract the patient by saying, "As soon as we finish in the bathroom, I'll get you a cookie." (or play Checkers, or some other enticement).

When accidents occur even using the timed voiding approach, or if the patient becomes ornery and resists every time you remind her to go, it is time for adult pull-up underwear. You don't want to trigger a huge power struggle every two hours, so if your loved one is strong-willed and refuses to go on a timed schedule—but then has an accident thirty minutes later—just surrender and invest in adult pull-ups.

Adult Pull-ups

Buy disposable pull-up underwear and buy them sooner rather than later. For cleanup, always have wet wipes and plastic bags available.

As a caretaker for two loved ones with Alzheimer's, I have dealt with more than my share of wet beds and adult disposable underwear. If I had to do it over, I would have started the disposable underwear earlier—much earlier!

Disposable pull-ups help prevent ruined mattresses, bedding, couches, car cushions, and clothing. They reduce the time you waste washing pants, and they prevent your home from smelling. Many people resist putting a loved one in pull-ups under the false notion that wearing a diaper is degrading. I waited a long time to use them on my mother and husband for that very reason. I wanted them to "keep their dignity" as long as possible.

When I finally got fed up with all the laundry and smell, I caved in and bought adult pull-ups. I expected a big fuss. "She'll never go along with it," I told myself. Imagine my shock when neither my mother nor my husband even noticed the difference between the cloth and disposable underwear. The problem had been mine.

~ If you only put disposable underwear in their dresser drawer, they will wear them without complaint. ~

Do not scrimp on adult pull-ups. Disposable underwear is essential to saving you time and energy. Pull-ups hold urine better and are easier to pull on and off since patients are already accustomed to pulling up their underwear. Adult pull-ups come in different sizes: small, medium, large, and extra-large. They also come in different absorbencies from moderate to super-plus. You might want to use medium during the day or in the car and super-plus at night.

Pull-ups still allow patients to use the bathroom—providing they can make it to the bathroom in time—but more importantly, they accommodate accidents, removing the worry that the patient will have an accident and ruin his trousers in public or soak the car upholstery. Pull-ups make it much easier to eat out in restaurants, visit people, take walks, run errands, go to church, and attend family outings without embarrassment or disruptive accidents.

Adult pull-ups can hold urine for three to four hours, which prevents the urine from irritating their skin if there is a delay getting home.

~ When taking your patient out for an extended period, put two adult pull-ups on—one on top of the other. That way, you won't have to remove the pants and shoes to make a diaper change. ~

~ The Two Pull-ups Procedure ~

1. **Have the patient stand.**
2. **Pull down the patient's pants or outer garment.**
3. **Pull down the clean outer pull-up.**
4. **Tear apart the soiled inner pull-up on the perforated sides and remove it front to back (to keep the wet part from touching the legs). Pulling front to back also reduces the risk of urinary tract infections.**
5. **Wipe the patient front to back with a wet one, and then pull the clean outer pull-up back up, followed by the patient's pants.**
6. **Place the soiled pull-up and wet one in a plastic bag, tie at the top, and drop in a trashcan.**

This quick and easy procedure keeps you from having to remove the patient's shoes and pants. Some people also use this system at night, especially if the loved one has to urinate frequently. After having your sleep interrupted three or four times a night, being able to change the pull-up quickly is critical This two pull-ups technique will allow you to make the diaper change quickly and get back to bed in under three minutes.

Dispose of soiled pull-ups in a plastic bag securely tied at the top. By securing it first in a plastic bag, you prevent odor issues. Ask your friends to save their plastic grocery bags, as you will need them.

When you are away from home, carry wet wipes and plastic bags in your purse or fanny pack. Keep them handy in the patient's bedroom and bathroom. Since public facilities aren't always private, a quick and easy cleanup is essential.

Even with disposable pull-ups, you will occasionally have an accident where the disposable underwear didn't hold. This is especially true in the later stages when the patient is no longer voiding independently at all. In my experience, accidents usually occurred at night or when we were away from home more than three hours.

Place extra pull-ups, trousers, and socks in a large tote bag that you keep in the trunk of your car. Carry the tote bag with you into the restaurant or social event, especially if you have to use a valet or park any distance away. Having a tote bag with a complete change of pants will keep you prepared for accidents.

Public Restrooms

When taking your patient with moderate or late-stage AD to a public restroom, he may require assistance. This can be an issue if you are helping someone of the opposite gender. Basically, there are three types of public restrooms: the family restroom; a unisex restroom; and the typical restroom identified as being for women or men. Ideally, the family bathroom is the best choice, but most establishments do not provide them.

If a store or restaurant has no family restroom, my personal choice is the handicapped stall of the lady's restroom because they are wider and accommodate two people better. It also provides complete privacy. As I brought my husband into the lady's restroom, I simply explained to the people in the restroom that my husband had dementia and needed assistance using the bathroom. Since I accompanied him into the bathroom and we were cloistered in a private handicapped stall, no one ever objected.

If the bathroom stall is too small for two people to fit in easily, you may have to stand with the stall door partially open, so that you can assist. Keep your husband unexposed as much as possible. If someone enters the bathroom, politely ask her to wait outside until you are finished so she won't get an eyeful. When she understands the reason, I always found people understanding and willing to wait.

Another option when out in public is to have your loved one wear two pull-ups using the technique described earlier. This can delay having to bring the patient into a public restroom at all.

I have two friends who took care of their wives in the latter stages of Alzheimer's, and they said they did not take them to public restrooms. They relied on pull-ups until they got home to avoid the awkwardness of having to go into women's restrooms.

Another friend, whose wife had a stroke and was wheelchair-dependent, solved the problem by stopping along the interstate at a nice hotel. He would go in and explain the situation and always found nice large wheelchair-accessible restrooms. He said the employees were always kind.

Come prepared with an extra change of clothes, wipes, diapers (if you are using diapers), and plastic bags in which to hold any soiled clothes. You may also want to bring a small can of air freshener like Febreze.

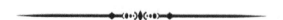

CHAPTER 17

─◆─‹•··›‹‹•·›─◆─

HOW TO KEEP PATIENTS ENTERTAINED
Sue Bell and Dr. Sally Burbank

One of the most exhausting parts of caring for patients with AD is figuring out how to keep them occupied during the day or how to protect them if they roam the house at night. While most retired people entertain themselves by reading, gardening, golfing, playing computer games, watching favorite TV programs, or participating in church activities and volunteer work, patients with AD progressively lose their ability to do many of these activities independently. Many doze in their recliners in front of the television for hours on end, or follow their caregiver around the house like a puppy. They may explore drawers, closets, or the refrigerator, leaving a mess that must be cleaned up. In late stage AD, they tend to sleep a lot and cannot do much of anything.

For patients with mild to moderately severe AD, the caregiver must direct the patient into activities that don't require much cognitive skill but will still keep them entertained and stimulated. Otherwise, the caregiver will not get much done.

First, consider your loved one's interests prior to AD and look for ways to alter that activity so they can still perform a simplified version. For example, while Ray was no longer able to play a full eighteen holes of golf, he still loved to go to the driving range or practice putting. Sometimes we would drive around the course in a golf cart.

Similarly, after Sally's father kept laying down runs that included both spades and clubs during a game of Rummy, the family changed the rules so a "run" didn't have to be one-suited—just all black or all red. By simplifying the rules, her father could still play a game he loved without getting frustrated.

We have listed below activities that appeal to many AD patients. Start with those that seem most attuned to your loved one's pre-AD interests.

AD Appropriate Activities

Jigsaw Puzzles: Use simple, large-piece puzzles. With the varying degrees of difficulty available, these can entertain patients until the last stage when even a four-piece puzzle will be challenging.

Building Blocks: Let them stack blocks high and then knock them over. Plastic containers with lids or Jenga game pieces can be used instead of real blocks. Clap and cheer to encourage them.

Lock a Block: This child's toy is a wooden box with all kinds of locks on it. You have to figure out how to lock and unlock each lock. Drawers come open once the lock is opened. Check on Amazon for similar locked box games.

Coloring Books: Adult coloring books have varying degrees of difficulty, or you may prefer to use children's books. As the disease progresses, the patient may need large crayons or magic markers. Some patients do better with large triangular crayons which are easier to grasp. These can be ordered online from a company called Melissa and Doug.

Jewelry Making/Arts and Crafts: Patients may enjoy stringing plastic, wood, or metal beads into necklaces that can be given as gifts to family members (who will understand if it looks like a child's arts-and-crafts project from summer camp). Supplies can be ordered online or at a hobby story such as Michael's or Hobby Lobby.

Magazines or Catalogs with lots of pictures: Choose the interests of your patient: golf, gardening, fishing, animals, birds, homes, cooking, tools, camping, etc. Check out picture books from the library of national parks or cookbooks with pictures of delicious desserts. Find the subject that interests the patient and keep the magazines and catalogs on a coffee table next to their favorite chair. Until his dying day, my father loved looking at seed and gardening catalogs even though he could no longer maintain a garden.

Golf: In early AD, Ray would hit golf balls on the driving range and putt. Sometimes I carried a chair and sat nearby reading my book. We also played miniature golf.

Simplified Home Golf: Place several wide-mouthed glasses on the floor and give your patient a putter and a Ping-Pong or golf ball. Let him try to get the ball into the cup. Provide cheers and encouragement when he succeeds. Like children, AD patients like to have their accomplishments acknowledged.

Tossing a Ball: While this has to be done with another person or with a dog, Ray loved to toss a ball back and forth. If you have a dog, Rover will be happy, too. This can also provide entertaining interaction with grandchildren and great-grandchildren.

Solitaire: In the beginning stages, most patients can still play Solitaire, so give them a deck of cards. Even in the middle stages, Ray would shuffle the cards and play the game incorrectly, but it kept him occupied!

Cards: When Solitaire becomes too challenging, have them try separating the cards into the four suits (spades, clubs, diamonds, and hearts); or separate them by numbers; or, using two or three decks, look for the Jokers and royalty cards. One caregiver shuffled three different packs of cards together and asked her mother to separate the cards into the three separate packs. As the disease progressed to late stage, she shuffled the three packs together and had her mother separate the red cards from the black cards. Write "RED" on an index card with a red crayon and "BLACK" with a black crayon and put them on the table as a reminder of where to put each color card. Sometimes they will forget what you told them to do, but the index cards will remind them. You can also challenge the patient to try to build houses or towns with the cards. It doesn't matter if they don't do the task correctly—the point is to keep your loved one entertained and challenged.

Yahtzee: This game has five dice. The patient is entertained as he rolls the dice and tries to come up with certain patterns. Direct him to shake the dice until he obtains ones on all five dice, then all twos, and so on. Or, you can play with him and help him know if he has a full house, four-of-a-kind, etc.

Family Photo Albums: Ask about a childhood picture while you fix dinner or fold laundry. This will trigger memories.

Funny Old Television Shows: "I Love Lucy," "The Andy Griffith Show," or "America's Funniest Home Videos." The language is simple and the facial expressions and antics entertaining.

Old Movies: An old cowboy movie would keep Ray entertained for an hour or so. He would also watch old musicals. Movies like *The Wizard of Oz* have amusing characters, and the music is soothing and familiar. The costumes and dancing are entertaining, even if the patient can't follow the plot. Also, these stories tend to have happy endings. Old movies can be borrowed from the library for free.

Favorite Television Programs: Channels like HGTV (Home and Garden) provide the opportunity to see an old beat-up house transformed into a showpiece or couples shopping for a new home. Ask the patient which of the three houses presented she would want to buy. What did she like best about it?

Nature or Travel Programs: The Planet Earth DVD series provides spectacular scenery and can be signed out from the library. PBS also has nature programs. While the patient won't understand or remember the dialog, the photography is stunning.

Yard Work: One AD patient enjoyed deadheading all the spent daisies, geraniums, and zinnias in her daughter's flower garden. The patient would go out with garden scissors early in the morning, before it got too hot, and tidy up all the plants. She also enjoyed watering them with a hose.

Laundry: AD patients can assist with separating whites from colors. They can match socks and fold underwear or T-shirts. Even if you have to re-do some of it, it keeps their hands busy.

Cooking: AD patients can assist with cooking. Let them beat the eggs, spread butter on the toast, or measure a cup of sugar from the canister. My father would husk the corn-on-the-cob and peel the potatoes. Flatten a roll of sugar cookie dough and let the patient enjoy using cookie cutters to shape cookies. Once they are baked, they can help frost them and apply sprinkles.

Loading the Dishwasher or Drying the Dishes: In early and middle AD, these are things the patient can do to help. They may be slow, but the job gets done.

Organizing Closets, Drawers, or Toolsheds: One woman had her mother organize all the shoes in her closet and then hang the clothes by color. She didn't do it correctly, but it kept her occupied for over an hour. Another man went to his toolshed and organized his tools for hours each day. Ask the patient to organize the junk drawer or a kitchen drawer that contains spatulas and wooden spoons.

Television: As the disease progresses, patients tend to spend more and more time watching television. With cable TV, you can find any genre of programming twenty-four hours a day: Westerns, home improvement, sports, golf, travel, old movies, family-friendly reruns, musicals, cooking shows, etc.

Warning! Most patients find non-stop CNN, Fox, or MSNBC news channels upsetting. Hearing incessant reports about terrorist attacks, bickering politicians, heroin epidemics, scandals, and the impending bankruptcy of Medicare and Social Security can be very troubling to patients. AD patients may become too agitated to sleep after listening to such reports. Avoid these channels at bedtime.

If your cable subscription includes Playboy or "adult" channels, take them off immediately! I have had a few caregivers tell me their demented fathers or husbands got addicted to porn channels when they were alone at night and couldn't sleep.

Bird Feeders: On bad weather days, I sat Ray down at the kitchen table and let him look out the window at the birds and squirrels. He would watch the rain and enjoy seeing birds at the feeder or flapping in the birdbath. I helped him fill the birdfeeder when it was empty. He enjoyed the delicate hummingbirds that frequented our red sugar-water feeder.

Make Bird Treats: Fill pinecones with peanut butter, roll them in birdseed, and then hang them from a tree near the window. For a less messy bird treat, string Cheerios and tie the string near a bird feeder. Baltimore orioles like slices of orange covered with grape jelly. You can also hang an overripe banana by its stem with the peel partially pulled away.

A Box of Stuff! I left two large boxes of random items in strategic places to keep Ray entertained at night. I put in hats, sunglasses, clothespins, old television remotes, kaleidoscopes, a cigar box with lots of trinkets inside, a large plastic storage box filled with progressively smaller plastic boxes. He would open them all and rummage through them as though they were Russian nesting dolls. In the smallest container, I packed a handful of goldfish crackers. Ray was up for several hours most nights, so this "explore" box kept him entertained while I slept. I would periodically change the items in the box.

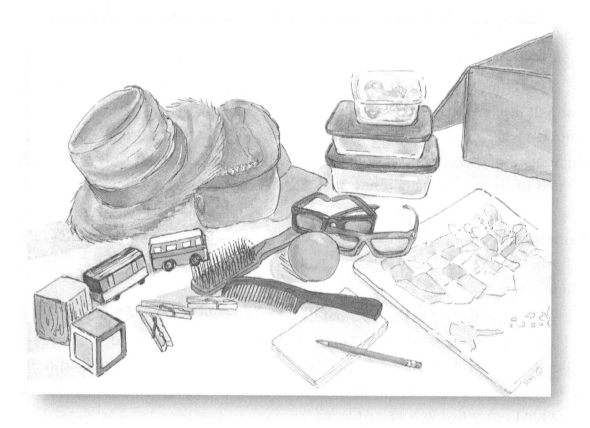

Rocking Chairs and Flowerbeds: Ray and I spent a lot of time on the front porch sipping coffee, especially in the early morning. He loved sitting on the porch enjoying the sunshine while I worked in the flowerbeds. While I deadheaded flowers and pulled weeds, I would keep up a running conversation describing the flowers I was planting. I would point out the neighbor's house and talk about the people who lived there. Conversing with him allowed me to work in the garden while keeping him safely nearby. I would tell him funny stories from our life together and talk about our kids and grandkids and what they were doing with their lives. Near the end, when he would no longer talk, I told him about his life and accomplishments—starting with college and continuing with his coaching days, years as a school principal and State Farm agent, and ending with his years as mayor of our town. I reminded him of people he had helped. This always brought a smile to his face. Sharing about our life together kept him entertained for several hours while I indulged my love of gardening. At the end, he didn't want me out of his sight, so he would sit in a lawn chair to watch me work. Early on, he could assist with the deadheading or weeding or mulching. By the end, he only watched.

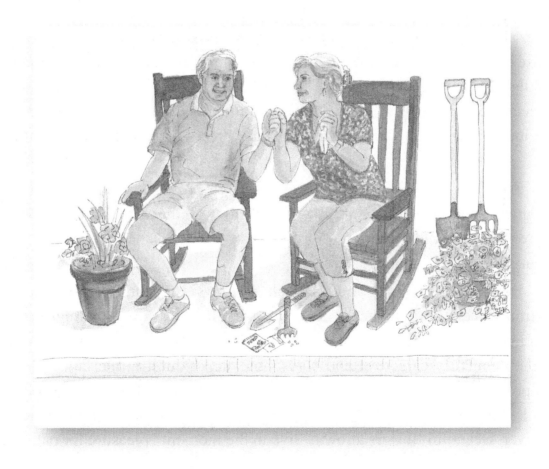

Crossword Puzzles, Word Searches, Where's Waldo? Books, Find These Items, and Easy Sudokus: Those who enjoyed brain challenges can continue to do so until fairly late in the disease. They may not get the right answers, especially as the disease progresses, but they will stay busy in their books. The challenge level can be decreased as the disease progresses.

Cleaning: One man said his wife loved to dust and mop the house. He would give her cleaning materials, and she would spend at least an hour each day dusting and tidying up the house. The house had never looked so good!

Tidying Up the Yard: One wife kept two large bushel barrels of sticks and trash in the garage. Before her husband with AD got up for the day, she sprinkled sticks, tree limbs, beer cans, and other litter all over the front yard. Since her husband had always taken great pride in his yard, he would spend over an hour every morning before breakfast, picking up the sticks and trash. He would often sputter about the "litterbugs," but the task provided exercise, something to do, and a sense of pride when the yard was tidy again. She praised him every morning over breakfast at what a great job he did keeping their yard looking nice. He seemed to appreciate feeling needed. While he worked in the yard, she could take a shower, get a load of wash done, and prepare a hearty breakfast—his favorite meal of the day.

Zoos: If there is a zoo anywhere nearby, it provides an ideal day trip. The AD patient, in a wheelchair if necessary, will enjoy all the animals. Season's passes are great, as they allow you to go for just an hour or two and then leave when the patient gets tired or cranky.

Botanical Gardens and Garden Centers: In Nashville, we have the beautiful Cheekwood Botanical Gardens. This makes a lovely outing to see the tulips in the spring, the coleus and perennials in all different colors in the summer, and the pumpkin, scarecrow, and chrysanthemum exhibit in the fall. A season's pass provides an incentive to get out of the house and stroll through beautiful flowers. Sunshine and fresh air is an instant mood elevator for both the patient and caregiver. Beautiful flowers allow a "live in the moment" pleasure for patients.

If you have no botanical garden nearby, visit a local nursery or Home Depot or Lowe's gardening center. Stroll through the aisles and ask your loved one which flowers or plants they most like. While this won't free you from your caregiving responsibilities, it will get you out of the house and around other people. Short day trips keep you from feeling trapped at home. As the disease advances, you may need to bring a wheelchair. Even if they say nothing, they will appreciate the sensory pleasure of colorful flowers.

Beanbag Toss: Line up a laundry basket, a Dutch oven, and a saucepan on the floor about eight feet from the patient. Have the patient try to toss a beanbag or small plastic ball into the three containers. Give one point for the laundry basket, three points for the Dutch oven, and five points for the saucepan.

Manicure/Pedicure: Even women with Alzheimer's enjoy pampering! Soak their hands and feet, massage them with moisture cream, and paint their nails with a favorite color of polish. Blow the nails dry with a hair dryer set on low. In the early stages, Mom can give you a foot or hand massage, as well.

Facial: Pamper Mom with a masque and then massage in a rich moisturizing cream. She'll love the attention.

Dolls: In the later stages of AD, some women enjoy dressing and undressing dolls. Some enjoy a favorite stuffed animal to talk to or dress, such as a "Build-a-Bear."

Arts and Crafts: Roam through a hobby store and you will find simple crafts your loved one can do. Pick up construction paper and multiple pairs of crimping scissors. Encourage the patient to make construction paper cards or tree ornaments.

Buttons: If you have a button box, let your loved one separate the buttons by color, or size, or into groups of five.

Singing: Lead your patient in singing, "Old McDonald Had a Farm" and come up with as many animals as she can. Other favorites include "Head and Shoulders, Knees and Toes" and "Jesus Loves Me." Even well into the late stage, most patients can remember the lyrics to old, familiar songs and hymns.

Dominos: Have the patient try to line up dominos on the table without knocking them down, then enjoy watching them fall.

Scrabble: Turn over all the letters and have the patient try to spell words on the board. Don't worry about counting points. You can also turn over the X, K, Q, and Z and make them extra blank letters that can be used as any letter they want.

Art Books: Check out books of art from the library that contain large colored prints of famous paintings. Provide the patient with Post-It Notes and ask her to mark the paintings she really likes. Later, you can have her show you her favorites. Ask why she likes them. You can do the same with picture books of dogs, flowers, African animals etc. The Post-It Notes provide something for her to do with her hands.

Make Gift Tags: Have the patient clip old greeting cards into gift tags, then punch a hole in the tag for the ribbon to go through.

Make Christmas Tree Ornaments: Help the patient mix four cups of flour, a cup of salt, and one-and-a-half cups of warm water. Knead the dough until smooth. Roll out to one-eighth-inch thickness. Let the patient use cookie cutters to cut out and place the ornaments on a cookie tray. Make a hole at the top of the ornament with a straw or blunted pencil. Bake 325 degrees for one hour. Help the patient paint the ornaments using non-toxic paint. Once the paint dries, pull a ribbon through the hole and hang on the tree. This home-made dough can also be used like Play-Doh.

Easter Eggs: Have the patient paint plastic Easter eggs to hang from an outdoor tree or fill the eggs with candy for an Easter egg hunt with the grandkids.

Clay or Play-Doh: Have the patient create things in different sizes and colors. Watch to make sure they don't eat it. Provide inspiration by displaying pictures of simple things they can try to make. As the disease progresses, they may just squish it in their fingers or make balls.

Jazzercise or Walking DVD: Even if the patient doesn't nail the dance steps, jazzercise or dance DVDs allow the patient and caregiver to get some exercise. Or, simply put on lively music and make up dance steps. The goal is to have fun and to get the patient moving. This is mostly appropriate for early and middle-stage AD.

Coupon Clipping: Using blunt-tipped scissors, have the patient clip coupons from the Sunday paper or from magazines.

Snow Sculptures or Snowmen: If you live in a snowy environment, take advantage of it and enjoy building and dressing a snowman or creating snow sculptures. Warning: AD patients might not be able to tell you when they are cold, so bundle up and don't stay out too long. Never leave them outside alone, or your loved one may wander off.

Bat at Balloons: Blow up a balloon and have fun volleying it back and forth. Make the goal to keep the balloon from touching the floor. Try a couple of balloons. Be aware a popping balloon sound may startle the patient.

Pair Socks: Have the patient try to match up pairs of socks. In the early stage, give her socks of different colors and sizes. In later stages, make the socks all identical black or white. Thank her for her help when all the socks are matched.

Letter Games: Brainstorm with the patient every word she can think of that begins with the letter P or B or L, etc.

Autumn Leaves Coasters: Help the patient find pretty autumn leaves in the yard. Sandwich the leaves between two pieces of waxed paper, top the waxed paper with a thin rag (to keep your iron clean), and iron on medium (without steam) to allow the wax on the paper to transfer to the surface of each leaf. Trim the edges into a circle to create coasters.

Flower Arranging: If you grow flowers, clip some with the patient and invite her to arrange the flowers in a vase.

Shredding Paper: Nancy L. kept her mother with moderate Alzheimer's entertained by having her feed documents into the shredder. Church members and family would all provide documents for her mother to shred. Since the caregiver worked as a nurse in a doctor's office, every Friday she brought home a box full of medical documents and paperwork requiring shredding. This freed the office receptionist from a time-consuming and dreaded task. Nancy paid her mother $5 an hour for her work. Her mother loved bragging to her friends that she was still working at age ninety.

Dried Flowers: Help the patient pick some violets, columbine, pansies, or other small flowers and lay them flat between 2 pieces of paper. Apply heavy books on top of the flowers for several weeks. Once the flowers are pressed, have the patient glue the flowers onto notecards or index cards.

Fly a Kite: On a windy day, go fly a kite with the grandkids or great-grandkids. Better yet, purchase a kite-making kit and have everyone help put it together first.

Tea Party: Arrange a tea party for the patient with a couple of her friends or the grandchildren or neighbors' children. Let her serve cookies on a pretty plate with a cup of tea.

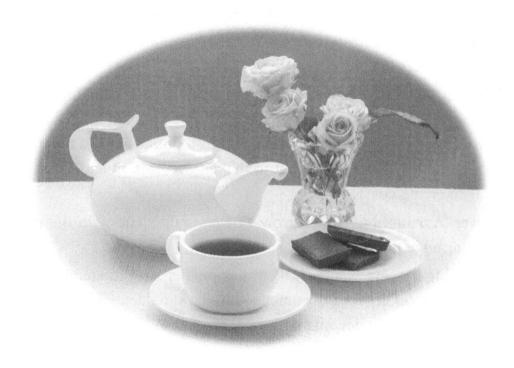

Pet Therapy

An affectionate cat or dog makes a fantastic playmate for a patient with AD for multiple reasons.

First, the cat or dog is often as bored as the AD patient and will love having someone pat them and throw balls to them. If you don't have a dog of your own, perhaps a neighbor would let the patient play fetch with theirs. You can tell your patient that the dog is bored and needs to be played with. This way, the patient feels like he is being helpful.

Second, pets provide unconditional love and affection. You don't have to have a fully functioning brain to stroke a friendly dog or enjoy the purr of a contented kitty in your lap.

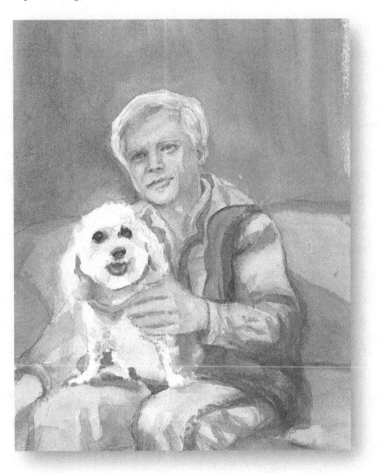

A fish tank filled with colorful goldfish is another low-maintenance option which can provide entertainment. Some stores even sell fish tanks with artificial fish that dive and dart like real ones. These can amuse late-stage AD patients.

Studies show people are calmer and happier after spending time with pets. Nursing homes and hospitals now allow volunteers to bring in dogs for patients to stroke and enjoy. In fact, the nursing home nearest Sue's house has a friendly cat that provides companionship for the residents.

If you don't currently have a pet, consider adopting a cat or dog from the Humane Society. Do not adopt a puppy or kitten, as they require a lot of work. I recommend a middle-aged cat or dog that is not too big; you don't want a large dog that knocks your loved one down! A short-haired dog will not require the brushing, bathing, or trips to a groomer that a long-haired breed might; you want the dog to be companion, not another time-consuming responsibility.

The Humane Society can assist in selecting a pet that is docile, friendly, and appropriate for the elderly. Do not pick previously abused animals, as the erratic behavior of an AD patient might trigger the dog to snap, bite, or growl. This could frighten your loved one.

A friendly cat may be a great alternative to a dog because they don't have to be walked and can be left alone for a weekend with a large bowl of food and a clean litter box. If you are dead set against owning a pet, consider this…

Many Humane Societies allow volunteers to pet cats or walk dogs. Most require a two-hour training session and would likely require the caregiver's participation, but this could be an ideal weekly activity to help an AD patient feel useful and provide love to a yet-to-be-adopted cat or dog. This could be presented to the patient as volunteer work to help the stray animals. Give the Humane Society a heads-up that your patient has memory issues, and perhaps ask the staff to thank the patient for his help each week. The patient might also bring a bag of pet food to present to the Humane Society as a donation.

Just because a patient has Alzheimer's, doesn't mean he loses his desire to feel useful. Loving on stray cats and dogs provides a perfect way for a memory-challenged person to "give back."

CHAPTER 18

EXPECT THE UNEXPECTED!
Sue Bell and Dr. Sally Burbank

You cannot imagine all the things your loved one will say and do as they navigate the stages of AD, nor is there a way to fully prepare yourself for the unexpected situations you will face. Most caregivers will tell you to have a plan, and then a backup plan. You may even need a backup plan for your backup plan!

My husband was a football player, and one of his favorite expressions when we got in a tight spot was, "I guess we'll have to punt." Be prepared to punt a lot. Not every plan you develop will gain yards on the field, much less a touchdown.

The first unexpected example I experienced came when Ray was in the middle stages of the disease. Ray was always generous and would give money to anyone who asked for it. As he was watching television one day, he came in the kitchen and said, "That woman said I was sick." Since we were the only two people at home, I did not know what he was talking about. I questioned him and after some checking, I realized he had called a psychic hotline. I was amazed because, by this time, I thought he was incapable of dialing the phone.

Another example: When dealing with Alzheimer's patients, many caregivers experience their loved ones not recognizing them. This is shocking the first time it happens, especially if you are around them all the time. I remember one day Ray asking me where his wife, Sue, was over and over. He would not believe that I was his wife! He kept saying, "She's dead, isn't she? You just don't want to tell me." I was shocked and hurt. It was hard not to cry.

During his later stages, I thought Ray no longer knew me. I realized this was not the case when I returned home after leaving him with a sitter and he smiled and acted very excited to see me. This helped me become aware that Ray did indeed recognize and miss me.

Other caregivers have learned to expect the unexpected. Here are examples:

- While riding home from church one Sunday, Everett W. said to his daughter, "I was so surprised to see my mother in church today." Since his mother had died thirty years earlier, his daughter asked, "Really? Where was she sitting?" He responded, "Right next to you." Turns out, he had confused his wife of sixty-five years with his dead mother. Later that day, when he was back in his familiar surroundings and had taken a nap, he recognized his spouse as his wife again.

- One AD patient called 911 insisting she was being held hostage by two strong men with guns and a ferocious dog. The dispatcher took the claim seriously, and a swat team rushed to her home. They swarmed around the house holding assault rifles prepared to rescue the hostage. Imagine the family's shock when the swat team barged through the front door and discovered no armed thugs or vicious dog—only a ninety-four-year-old AD patient who had awakened from a nightmare unable to differentiate her dream from reality. Somehow, she had rallied enough memory to dial 911. As you can imagine, the swat team was amused (and relieved, no doubt), but the family was mortified.

- John D. was brought to his son's house for a few days while his wife had minor surgery. John D. did not recognize or seem to know who his son was, but he sat at the table and talked with him for two hours. The subject? How much he loved his son and how proud he was of him. Just imagine how touched and pleased the son was to hear all the memories his father had of him!

- John D.'s family had disconnected the battery from his car and removed it, so he could no longer drive the vehicle. One day, however, he found the hidden battery, hooked it back up, and drove away!

- Mary E. had taken her father's car keys in order to keep him from driving. One day he said to a sitter who had been hired to stay with him, "I can't find my car keys anywhere, but if you go into the garage and look under the bucket of nails on the shelf, I have a spare hidden there. Let's go for a ride." Sure enough, the sitter found the spare key hidden under a bucket of nails, just as he said.

- Danny D. slept in a recliner instead of the bed. One night, he asked his wife if he could sleep in the bed with her. She replied, "Sure." When she later found him back in his chair, she said, "I thought you were going to sleep in the bed with me." Danny D. replied, "No, it wouldn't be right." He obviously didn't recognize her as his wife.

- Sometimes the unexpected situation can be a pleasant surprise. Patsy B. went to visit a friend with Alzheimer's disease. The friend hadn't recognized her in months and normally didn't say much, but this day when Patsy asked her friend, "Do you know who I am?" Her friend responded, "Of course! You're Patsy." Patsy was shocked.

Moral of the story? Be prepared for anything!

Sense of Humor

We've all heard the adage by Greek philosopher Epictetus, "It's not what happens to you, but how you react to it that matters." Since Alzheimer's patients can react in unusual and embarrassing ways, maintaining a sense of humor will help you keep your sanity. Far better to laugh than to cry, right?

Ray had gotten to the point where he would forget to tie his shoelaces. My daughter Cindy was looking for a Father's Day gift and thought slip-on shoes would be perfect, so we took him to a local shoe store. Ray did not want to get out of the car, so she went into the store and brought out a shoe in his size to try on. Meanwhile, I stayed in the store looking at the different styles.

Cindy came back into the store to tell me the shoe was way too small. "He needs something much larger," she insisted.

I argued with her. "Ray has always worn a size nine."

She shrugged. "I'm telling you, it didn't fit."

Unconvinced, I grabbed the shoe and marched back to the car to see for myself. When I pulled up his pant leg and looked at his feet, they were huge! *What on earth?* Had he developed massive swelling overnight? I bent down to inspect further and discovered he had on more than one sock. I took off the first pair of socks and discovered another pair. And then another! All told, I pulled off a total of five pairs of socks.

The sales clerk stood watching, and I remember thinking, "She must think I'm a terrible caregiver."

Luckily, the clerk chuckled. "Don't worry, I understand. My grandfather had Alzheimer's."

I looked over at the stack of socks and burst into laughter. *Five pairs of socks! Good grief!* We all cracked up, including Ray! Why? Better to choose humor over humiliation.

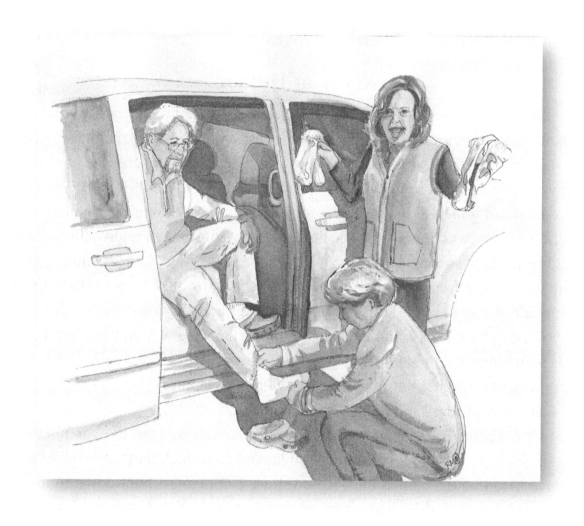

More Unexpected Behaviors

- Arlene P. had reached the stage in her Alzheimer's where she was no longer verbal. One day, while sitting at the table with her daughter Janie, she picked up the vase of daisies in the center of the table, removed the flowers, and began drinking the vase water. She was obviously thirsty but lacked the verbal and non-verbal ability to communicate that she needed a glass of water. Interestingly, she was still able to problem-solve enough to quench her thirst, but she lacked the judgment to recognize vase water was inappropriate. After that, the family made sure glasses of water were readily available throughout the house, so Arlene wouldn't resort to drinking vase water.

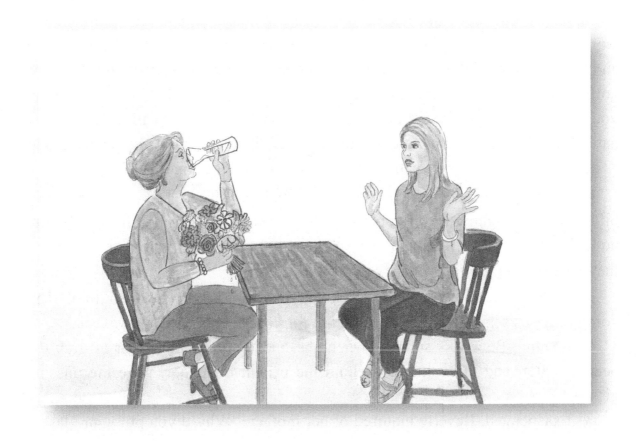

- Ray, in the later stages, loved to shake hands with people whether he knew them or not. At one point, he started telling everyone, "I sure do love you." Around family and close friends this was not a problem. But one day, we were in the grocery store, and he walked up to an elderly woman, shook her hand, and said, "I sure do love you."

She turned to me and snapped, "What do you think about that?"

I was stunned at her reaction. Before I could reply, she stormed off. I had a choice: I could either dwell on the woman's reaction and my embarrassment, or I could make the choice to find humor in the situation. Since no real harm had occurred, I made the choice to not let it ruin my day. After all, Ray didn't mean to embarrass me.

- A minister came to visit Nora S. in the nursing home. When he entered the room, she asked him to take his hat off. "I'm not wearing a hat," he informed her. Nora insisted he was wearing a hat, so the minister pantomimed taking off his hat and hanging it on the hook on the back of the door. After a long chat with Nora, he got up to leave and pretended to pick up a hat and put it on his head. "What are you doing?" Nora inquired, a puzzled expression on her face. "I'm putting on my hat before I leave," he said. After the minister left the room, Nora told her daughter, "There's something wrong with that man. He didn't have a hat!"

- Mary, an elderly patient with AD, had misplaced her expensive new bifocals. Her daughter, Beverly, performed an exhaustive search of the house with no luck. Mary had not left the house since the last time she'd worn her glasses, so they had to be in the house somewhere. But where?

After a full hour of futile searching, Beverly gave up in frustration. "I'm going to fix us some lunch. We can search for your eyeglasses after we eat."

Imagine Beverly's surprise when she opened the pantry door to grab the peanut butter, and there, hidden behind the peanut butter jar, were the missing glasses!

Exasperated, Beverly inquired of her mother, "Why'd you put your glasses in the pantry?"

Mary shrugged and made up an excuse. "I guess I didn't want 'em stolen. I must've put 'em in the pantry 'cause no thief would look for them there."

Beverly shared this story with me with a smile on her face. Like most successful caregivers, she'd learned to appreciate the humor of her mother's antics.

- Margaret L. was convinced someone had stolen her coat. Her daughter helped look for it and eventually found it in the closet. Upon seeing the coat, Margaret scowled. "They stole my good white coat and left me with this worn-out yellowed one." It was actually Margaret's ten-year-old coat, but she remembered it the way it looked when she bought it.

In summary, you don't have a choice about a lot of things when you care for someone with Alzheimer's, but you can choose how you react. Find the humor whenever possible, and you will mentally fare much better.

CHAPTER 19

THE STIGMA OF ALZHEIMER'S

Dr. Sally Burbank & Sue Bell

Unfortunately, there is a stigma associated with Alzheimer's disease. When someone is first diagnosed with it, people often talk in hushed tones, as though the disease were something to be ashamed of. They also start treating the patient differently, something patients with early Alzheimer's find demeaning. Acquaintances talk louder as though the patient were deaf, or they dumb down their words as though talking to a six-year-old. "I may have trouble remembering, but I'm not stupid," one frustrated early AD patient told me at his yearly exam.

Perhaps the most upsetting thing Alzheimer's patients experience is the tendency of people to talk to the spouse but ignore the patient altogether. "My wife and my daughter will talk about me as though I'm not even in the room. Don't I get a say about anything?"

Throughout history, many other diseases carried a stigma: polio, cancer, tuberculosis, and AIDS, to name a few. Gradually, as the scientific basis of these diseases became understood and the general public became better educated, the stigma lifted. But we're not quite there with Alzheimer's.

Dealing with Public Opinion

When Ray was alive, people asked me how he was doing in a whisper, as though his condition were some kind of shameful family secret. Because of this, many patients and family members are reluctant to acknowledge the disease in public, even when it starts to become obvious.

Especially in early AD, the individual still holds a lifetime of experience and wisdom. He may retain a breadth of knowledge about his field of study, but all of this may be dismissed with a flippant, "He doesn't know anything… he has Alzheimer's." Uninformed friends and family often assume that a person with AD has suddenly become stupid.

In reality, AD is a slowly progressive disease, and in early AD, the patient retains most of their cognitive function. Gossips, however, seemed to delight in divulging, "Did you know Ray Bell has Alzheimer's?" with the same tone they might use to inform you he had had an affair or molested a child! This cruel tendency causes heartache and turmoil for patients and families alike.

I first recognized the social stigma of AD when a lady in town told me her husband said if he ever got demented, he didn't want to be dragged around town for everyone to gawk at and gossip about. She realized later her comment was rude, as I was sitting in the restaurant with Ray at the time! She later called to apologize.

Her comment made me ask myself, however, "Am I doing the right thing when I take Ray out every day and expose him to public ridicule? Are the caregivers who keep their loved ones tucked away at home—thereby protecting their reputation—doing the right thing?"

People came up to me showing concern for Ray, but after this lady's comment, I wondered, "What do people really think? Are they truly concerned, or do they go home and secretly think I shouldn't be exposing him to public scrutiny in his condition?" Ray had been a highly intelligent community leader—our town mayor, in fact. Was I marring his previously stellar reputation with my choice?

After much reflection and prayer, I decided I wouldn't have much of a life if I kept Ray home all the time. I enjoyed getting out, and so did Ray. He had always been a people person, so it wouldn't be good for either of us to stay isolated. How could I maintain my mental health if I was trapped home all the time with someone who wasn't capable of engaging in normal conversation?

Thus, I decided I would not let my life be dictated by the worry of what other people thought or said about me. I hope this book will motivate other caregivers to be brave enough to live life fully and not be controlled by the fear of what other people may think and say. The people who matter most will understand and support you. The rest have not walked in your shoes and may never understand.

CHAPTER 20

INAPPROPRIATE AND ANNOYING BEHAVIORS
Sue Bell and Dr. Sally Burbank

After giving you a pep talk to get out in public with your AD patient, I should now caution you there is a price to be paid. Namely, AD patients can sometimes behave in peculiar and inappropriate ways. At some point your loved one will say or do something to embarrass you, as in, "I-want-to-crawl-under-the-table-and-never-come-out" embarrassment. As a result, some caregivers quit going out. But a change in scenery is beneficial for both patient and caregiver, so go ahead—have a life. Just be prepared to handle inappropriate comments or strange behaviors.

Inappropriate behaviors may include...

- Talking to strangers as if they were long-lost friends.
- Interacting with children without sensing it makes the child and parents uncomfortable.
- Not understanding how to pay for things properly.
- Shoplifting.
- Eating with their fingers instead of with a utensil.
- Putting non-food items in their mouth.
- Wandering away from their caregiver.
- Making offensive or weird comments.
- Going into the wrong gender restroom.
- Getting lost in a restaurant on the way back from the restroom.
- Having a public meltdown with shouting or crying when they get upset or agitated.

- Cursing in public.
- Touching or fondling their genitals.

Most caregivers are selective about where they go due to the impulsive nature of the patient's comments and behaviors. Choose places like Senior Citizen lunches where others will be tolerant and understanding, or patronize familiar establishments, so the staff becomes familiar with your loved one.

When you go to a restaurant, be proactive and run interference to avoid a scene. AD patients often cannot sit still, so you would be wise to select a restaurant that takes reservations or doesn't have significant wait times. If allowed, call and place your order ahead of time. As the disease progresses, you will want to order for the patient to avoid embarrassment or wasting the server's time. If the patient tends to get restless, provide crayons and paper to keep him entertained while you wait for your meal.

As you enter the restaurant, hold the patient's arm and talk to him. This will distract him as you head toward your table. If you have a large group, surround your loved one until you reach your table. Otherwise, many dementia patients will

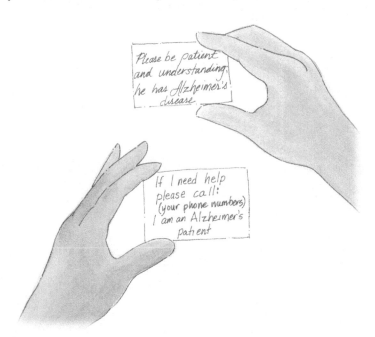

want to interact with other patrons, even though they are strangers. If you cannot keep your loved one from stopping to chat, simply smile and whisper discretely to the other party, "I'm sorry, he has dementia," and move on, or hand them a note that says, "He has dementia. Thanks for your patience." Most people, once informed, are kind and understanding.

In the grocery store, let the patient push the shopping cart. This distracts him by giving him a job to do. It also keeps him from wandering away or putting items in the cart that you don't want. Just be careful he doesn't bash into someone.

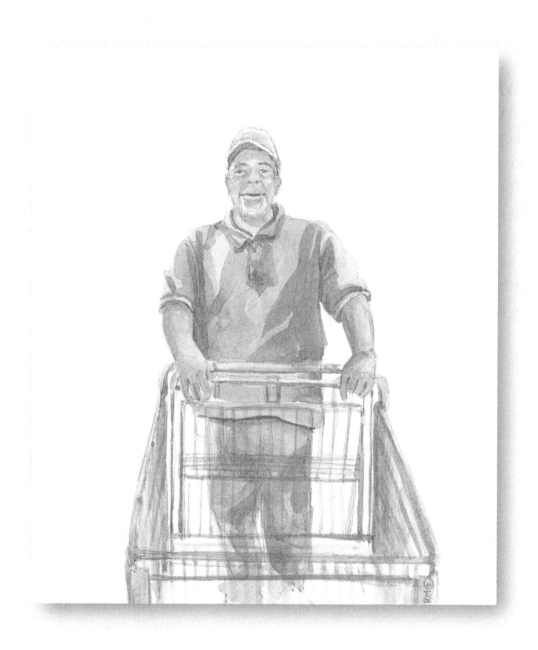

Dementia patients seem drawn to children, which can make the child or the child's parent uncomfortable. Perhaps the happy, carefree nature of children appeals to Alzheimer's patients. Unfortunately, when the dementia patient tries to interact with little ones, it often scares them. Again, be proactive. Calmly redirect the patient away from the child by pointing at something, then take his hand and escort him in that direction. If this doesn't work, stay close and explain the situation to the child and parent. Children may not understand dementia, but you can tell them that the patient has a condition that makes him act funny or get confused. Or, you can tell the child your AD patient loves his grandchildren and thought the child was one of his grandkids. Then move away as quickly as possible. Smile and wave good-bye to the child to reinforce that the AD patient is harmless.

Some caregivers carry index cards with the words, "Please be patient and understanding. He has Alzheimer's disease." These can be subtly handed to a parent to help explain your loved one's odd behavior without embarrassment.

The joy children bring a dementia patient is demonstrated in the following story:

One patient was riding in a car with his daughter and her three boisterous young boys. She was afraid their loud noise was bothering him. When she started reprimanding the boys for being too loud, her father reached over and touched her hand. He then touched his heart and said, "Happy right here." She realized that the laughter and fun coming from the back seat was not bothering him. In fact, he was enjoying their banter.

Public Behaviors that Aren't Easy to Excuse

- Lily M. and her husband were eating at a restaurant when a morbidly obese woman waddled by their table. Lily M. popped the lady on her backside with her hand and commented loudly to her husband, "She sure is a big one, isn't she?" The woman turned around and glared at the husband thinking he had made a pass at her. Talk about embarrassing!

- Laura P. would drop her mother off at the hair salon with enough money to cover a shampoo, style, and tip. While her mother got her hair worked on, Laura would run to the store for her weekly groceries. One week, when Laura called to schedule her mother's hair appointment, the stylist said, "I can't keep fixing your mother's hair for a dollar." That is all she had been paying the hairdresser! Her mother was clearly stuck in a gone by era when a haircut only cost a dollar. Mortified, Laura paid the hair stylist for all the previous haircuts—plus tips!

• Inappropriate behaviors can happen at home, too. Mary C.'s husband started urinating in inappropriate places: the potted plants, the umbrella holder, the pantry. She realized, after keeping a journal, that this happened when she was talking on the telephone. From then on, she made sure she only talked on the phone at length when he was asleep. The problem disappeared.

• Mary M. lived in a nursing home and several times got out of bed, wandered down the hall, and climbed into the bed of a male patient. This man, understandably, was startled when he woke up with a stranger in his bed! The family was convinced she thought she was in bed with her husband who had died several years earlier.

• Karen S. would sometimes catch her father touching his genitals when other people were in the room. Thankfully, he never exposed himself, but his behavior made everyone extremely uncomfortable. Karen learned to nonchalantly walk over to her father, lift his hand and whisper, "Don't touch there in front of other people. It makes them uncomfortable." She would then give him something to hold such as a Rubik cube. She discovered he tended to do this when he needed to urinate.

• If inappropriate touching or undressing become a problem, purchase or make an "activity apron" which is worn over the clothes. It has zippers, ribbons, buttons, a key ring with keys, and other notions attached to keep the patient's hands busy. These can be purchased online from Amazon.

Horrible Treatment of Sitters and Aides

One of the most exasperating behaviors caregivers deal with is the overt rudeness AD patients can display to sitters and home health aides hired to watch or give in-home care.

The worst case I learned about was a retired farmer who threatened to shoot the sitter his wife had hired while she attended a weekend church retreat. Before leaving for the weekend, the wife needed to run to the store to pick up a few items, so she forewarned her husband that someone might come to the house while she was out. "I'll be back in twenty minutes," she reassured him.

The poor sitter innocently rang the doorbell, and after introducing herself, was greeted by the barrel of a shotgun and a threatening voice hollering for her to get off his property or he'd fill her #$%& behind with buckshot. He didn't have to ask twice—she got out of there lickety-split! The farmer's wife had to forego the church retreat because she now had no one to watch her husband. When she asked him why he threatened to shoot the sitter, he simply said he didn't know her and thought she was an intruder. This brings me to some important advice:

~ Always be there when an AD patient meets a new caregiver, and never rely on the patient's memory to remember what you tell him. ~

The story also brings up another point: Guns are not safe in the home of Alzheimer's patients. The sitter could easily have been shot before the wife returned from the store.

When hiring a new sitter, set aside an hour or so to observe the interactions between the new caregiver and the patient. A sitter who is inflexible, argumentative, impatient, or bossy will not be a good match and could trigger horrible behavior. Also, never use the word "sitter" in front of the patient. Instead, call her "our new friend." Make sure she has experience with dementia patients and not just elderly people in general, as caring for AD patients requires a different skill set.

Sitters who are overly controlling or shaming may end up with food flung in their face as well as hitting, biting, yelling, or spitting. Warn the sitter of any previous triggers you have discovered that set the patient off. Reiterate that if the patient doesn't want to do something, don't force it—it usually backfires. Instead, the sitter should distract the patient and then come back to what she wanted him to do after a few minutes have passed. The sitter should always use an enthusiastic tone, plenty of patience, and perhaps even a cookie bribe. If a caregiver or volunteer sitter has never sat with an AD patient, you will need to educate them using the advice in this chapter.

Once you find a caregiver who gets along with your loved one, treat the sitter like a jewel—because she is one. Make sure to pay her well. If she refuses money, provide gift cards, thank you notes, verbal praise, or delicious baked goods— anything to make her want to come back. Reliable and caring sitters are your greatest treasure. Do not take these angels for granted.

A note of caution: Whenever you bring a new worker into your home, be sure to keep expensive jewelry, silver, and other valuables locked up. Checkbooks, controlled medications (i.e. pain pills), credit cards, and cash should be secured— not left lying in a drawer or cabinet. My family once lost an antique diamond ring not long after my parents hired workers to paint the room where my mother kept her jewelry.

Mean Comments

The frontal lobe of the brain is responsible for discernment and impulse control. A fully-functioning frontal lobe in the brain of a healthy person will filter that person's thoughts and make him or her think twice before blurting out inappropriate comments or acting in ways they will regret. This, unfortunately, is

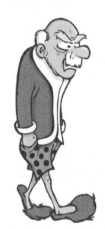

the very area of the brain where Alzheimer's disease causes shrinkage and progressive dysfunction. As a result, when a patient cannot do all the things he once could, he gets frustrated, and because he lacks the ability to articulate these feelings, he may lash out with unfiltered comments.

He may resort to swearing or using vulgar language. He may blurt out that you are too fat, or wearing an ugly dress, or that you have a huge nose. Even worse, he may threaten you or accuse you of stealing.

When a neighbor came for a visit, one AD patient nearly clobbered him with a baseball bat because he no longer recognized the neighbor and thought he was an intruder.

So what can you do when your loved one makes cruel comments?

First, remind yourself the patient would never act this way if he had a healthy brain. If the patient makes a rude comment to someone who has cooked him a nice breakfast, such as, "I can't eat this—the bacon is tough, and the eggs are burnt," you will have to do damage control. "I'm sorry. He has dementia and doesn't mean to be rude." Then try to find the humor. "Guess you won't be serving him bacon and eggs again. Cold cereal for him it is!"

Second, ask the patient's doctor if any of the medications could be exacerbating the problem; some medications cause personality changes.

Third, keep a journal of the situations that trigger temper tantrums or verbal outbursts. Over time, you may be able to pinpoint and avoid the triggers that cause your loved one to act up. Often fatigue, fear, frustration, and overstimulation are to blame.

Thankfully, because of their poor memories, patients quickly forget about their emotional outbursts. They have a childlike mentality and may speak with no thought about the feelings of the listener. They may tell you they hate you because you insist they take a bath, but ten minutes later, they will be perfectly fine with no recollection of their hateful words.

Unfortunately, it will be far harder for *you* to not dwell on the cruel comments. Even though you know Mom has a brain disorder and can't help it, her mean words hurt, especially when you are wearing yourself out caring for her.

- Perhaps the cruelest comment came from an Alzheimer's patient who told her caregiving daughter—whose sister had died five years earlier—that "the wrong daughter died." The "wrong" daughter, who happened to be fixing her mother's hair at the time, forced herself to reply calmly, "I'm sorry you feel that way, Mom. I miss Jenny, too." She continued fixing her mother's hair, but when she was finished, she left the room and sobbed. The cruel comment cut like a knife.

- Another example happened to a wife who was tending to her husband. In the early stages of his disease, he was frustrated at not being able to do all the things he used to do. One day, after his wife had to help him with a mundane task, he lashed out. "You think you know everything, and that I'm dumb!" Rather than fight back, she calmly responded, "No, you're actually very smart. You just have a memory problem, that's all." He calmed down and replied, "I feel like I can't do anything anymore. Thank you for saying that."

Getting past a hurtful comment is difficult, but necessary. It may help to keep a list of kind words or deeds from the past to remind yourself who your loved one was prior to AD.

How should you respond to a cruel comment?

- **Maintain a quiet, kind voice.** Speak with a smile on your face, even if the smile is forced. Never argue, contradict, or hurl something ugly back. Many times, the patient will respond to your body language. Your smile, touch, and kindness can change her behavior. You can calmly tell her the comment hurt your feelings, though she probably won't apologize. Take a time-out so you can calm down. Cry if necessary. When you return to the room, change the subject or distract the patient with something pleasant. Resist the urge to retaliate with a mean comment of your own, or the situation may escalate.

- **Vent to a trusted friend or family member.** You don't have to bottle up your hurt and anger—just don't retaliate on a person who no longer has the cognitive skills to understand her egregious behavior. I once had a close friend whose nerves were so frayed by her exasperating father that she called me up and sputtered, "My father isn't going to die of Alzheimer's… I'm going to kill him first!" She felt safe venting her feelings to me because she knew I understood how difficult caring for an impossible person like her father could be. (He had just taken a meal she had lovingly prepared and dumped it all over the floor, saying, "I don't want spaghetti!") Yes, in that moment of frustration, she wanted to wring his neck, but she also recognized that her father's brain was not functioning in a normal way.

- **Join an Alzheimer's support group.** If there isn't one in your community, consider starting one, or join an online support or Facebook group of caregivers. Your local chapter of the Alzheimer's Association should be able to assist you in finding a safe place to vent.

- **Forgive yourself if you hurl an ugly comment.** We're all human, and AD patients can push our buttons. Recognize you are most likely to lose it with your loved one when you are tired and need a break. Go outside, sit on the porch, take slow deep breaths, or take a short walk until you calm down. Remind yourself that your loved one will have forgotten your ugly retort by morning. You will not damage the patient's self-esteem long term if you occasionally lose your cool and say something ugly.

Repetitive Comments

One of the most annoying issues that families have to tolerate is the tendency of AD patients to repeat phrases, questions, or stories over and over. And over!

Why do they do this?

First, they don't remember telling you their story earlier, and they don't remember the answer you provided to their question, so they have to ask again.

Second, the brain malfunction of AD can make a particular question or comment get stuck in their head like a broken record.

How should you handle this? See if you can uncover the emotion or unmet need behind the repetitive question. Since AD patients can't verbalize what they are feeling or wanting in a more direct manner, they fixate on a question.

For example, if the patient keeps asking you what time it is, he may really mean, "I'm bored," "I'm hungry," or, "I'm nervous about the doctor's appointment this afternoon." Instead of answering for the tenth time, "It's eleven o'clock," try asking, "Why do you ask? Are you feeling restless? Let's find something fun to do," or "How about I get you a snack to tide you over until lunch," or "I'll bet you're feeling anxious about seeing Dr. Collins today." Once the need is met, they will often drop the question.

Another common repetitive statement is, "I want to go home." Patients may say this even when they are in their own house. This usually means they feel insecure. Try giving them a hug and reassuring them, "I'm going to take good care of you no matter where you are." If that fails, try, "What do you remember most about your home?" They may then describe their childhood home or the way their house looked before you bought new carpet and a flat screen TV. If you can get them to talk about the home they remember, it may calm them down. If not, try distraction and delay. "Let's have a snack before we go home."

Another common question is, "Where is my wife?" or "Where's Sue?" even if you are right there with him! Questions like these mean the patient is feeling insecure and afraid of abandonment because he no longer recognizes you as his wife. In his mind, his wife has disappeared, and some stranger has taken her place. It is pointless to tell him, "I am Sue," or, "I am your wife," because he won't believe you. A better response is, "Your wife asked me to take good care of you until she gets back. How about I pull out a scrapbook, and we can look at pictures of your Mama and Daddy," or "How about we play a game of checkers until Sue gets back?" In short, after you reassure him he is not abandoned, try distracting him with something comforting, enjoyable, and familiar.

Distraction works. Try asking him a question to get his mind on something different. You can point at something in the room or outside the window and start talking about it in a calm voice. "It is supposed to snow today. Did you ever play in the snow as a kid?" Or try singing a favorite hymn.

Humor works wonders. To lighten the mood, one caregiver made up a silly jingle. When the patient kept asking, "What time is my doctor's appointment?" she answered in singsong: "The doctor wants to see you at ten, so have your checkbook, purse, and pen." What the patient really needed, of course, was reassurance that the doctor's appointment would go okay.

• Arlene P. was going on a vacation to the mountains with her family. For weeks before the trip, she kept parroting, "Going to the mountains, going to the mountains …" She was "stuck" on this comment like a broken record. Her family provided her with a book of colorful wildflowers and birds she might see on the trip in hopes of distracting her. It only worked slightly, and she was soon back to parroting, "Going to the mountains." By the day of the trip, the family wanted to stuff a sock in her mouth! Thankfully, once the trip was over, she no longer made the annoying mountain comment.

~ Don't tell AD patients about upcoming trips or appointments until the day of the trip. Otherwise, they may obsess, stew, and ruminate, because they have no sense of time. ~

- Once she got back from the mountains, Arlene got stuck on the name of one of her daughters: "Vicki, Vicki, Vicki ..." Vicki herself needed fulltime care due to a physical disability, and the family suspected their mother was worried about who would provide that care after she died. Their mother was no longer capable of discussing her worries, so she expressed her fear in the only way she knew how— repeating Vicki's name. Vicki's siblings assured their mother repeatedly that they would always take care of Vicki. Eventually, Arlene stopped parroting Vicki's name.

~ Look for the underlying worry behind a repetitive comment and then reassure the patient. ~

- One exasperated caregiver snapped at her demented mother, "You've already asked me that question a hundred times." The patient responded, "I don't mind asking again if you don't mind answering."

- Another caregiver found giving her mother chewing gum or candy distracted her and kept her mouth busy.

- One particularly trying day, when I had not handled Ray's repetitive comments as well as I should have, I went to bed stewing about my impatience. That night, I had a vivid dream that has stuck with me, and it helped me in the challenging days that came ahead. In my dream, someone said to me, "Don't criticize a bird for singing the only song he knows."

Don't criticize a bird for singing the only song he knows.

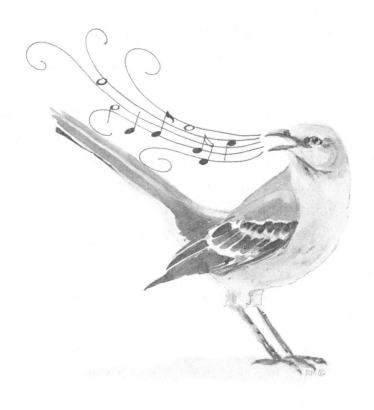

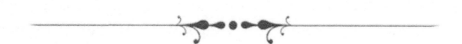

Nightmares or Bizarre Dreams

Night seems to be the worst time for AD patients. They wake up with strange dreams or nightmares and become confused and frightened because their ability to separate the dream from real life is hindered.

When your loved one has an upsetting dream, here are some ways to help calm them down:

- Turn on the lights and take the patient out of the bedroom.
- Use a calm, soothing voice, hold her hand, walk around the house to demonstrate there are no wolves or people chasing her or rivers drowning her. Explain that when we sleep, we experience dreams that are like miniature movies. They seem real, but they are not.
- Talk about a happy memory from their childhood.
- Look at a catalog or magazine together.
- Turn on a favorite movie or soft music.
- Ask about their favorite foods.
- Make a snack together.
- Talk about a favorite hobby or sort through a bowl of colorful buttons and look for a matching pair.
- Pull out a large-piece, simple jigsaw puzzle and work it with the patient.
- Ask about a sports game they would like to attend.
- Look through picture books of national parks or beautiful places around the world. Ask the patient which ones they would like to visit.

~ Remember: Distraction, distraction, distraction! ~

Making Messes and Snooping Around

In the fifteen minutes it takes for you to shower, your loved one can paw through every drawer and closet in your bedroom leaving a mess for you to pick up. In fact, exploring cabinets, drawers, and boxes is a favorite pastime for patients.

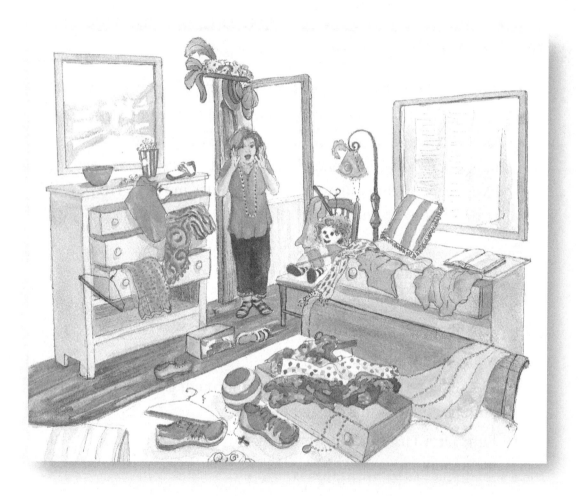

While caregivers find their loved one's snoopy behavior vexing, a teenager in the home can feel especially violated. "Can't you keep Grandma from pawing through my stuff?" they complain. Teens have been known to position a chair in front of their bedroom door to act as a barricade while at school. Baby latches can help, or a large red stop sign on the door may serve as a reminder to stay out. One frustrated teen even resorted to stretching duct tape across his door to act as a deterrent.

Keep valuables and family heirlooms locked up or in a safe deposit box, because Grandma may squirrel them away and forget where she put them.

Always scan the contents of waste baskets before dumping them, as your loved one may have thrown something valuable away, such as silverware, dentures, knickknacks, keys, and remote controls. Speaking of remote controls …

Where's the remote?

A caregiver can waste an inordinate amount of time looking for items that AD patients misplace. Adding insult to injury, the patient may turn around and accuse you of misplacing or stealing their stuff! Eyeglasses, dentures, house keys, money, the remote control … they all have a way of disappearing.

One thing you can do to help is put a large, colorful basket next to the patient's favorite chair, and label the basket in bold letters "Keys, Remote Control, Glasses" or whatever they commonly misplace. Tape a picture of each item to the basket, as well. By being easily accessible—in plain sight and clearly labeled—they may begin to put their stuff in the basket. You may also want to put bright orange stickers on the remote to make it easier to see.

Common hidey-holes include the pantry, the refrigerator, an underwear or sock drawer, under or in a mattress (especially money), under the couch cushions, or between towels in the linen closet.

AD patients are notorious for hiding money, fearing it will be stolen from their purse or wallet. Then they don't remember stashing it, and they may accuse you of stealing it. More than one caregiver has told me they discovered stashes of money long after their AD patient had died—under a jar of pickles, stuffed in a bag of winter mittens, in the back of a closet, and in a shoe. Jewelry is frequently squirreled away in bizarre places, so lock up anything expensive, and only allow the patient to have a few dollars at a time in their purse or wallet if they are prone to hiding and losing things.

Shadowing

One of the biggest complaints I hear from caregivers is that their loved one follows them around the house like a puppy. In fact, the patient gets addled if the caregiver is out of their sight for more than a few minutes.

One upset patient, Vernon, called his son and claimed his wife, Myrleen, had left him alone for "a very long time" and hadn't told him where she was going. The son tried calling his mother on her cell phone, but she didn't answer. Worried something terrible had happened, he left work and dashed to his parents' house. Imagine his shock—and relief—when he found Myrleen in the kitchen calmly making pancakes. She had been in the bathroom taking a long bath when her son called.

"I told you I was going to take a bath," she sputtered at Vernon. "You didn't need to pester our son at work. I was right here."

The son was understandably aggravated over leaving work for nothing. Mom was upset that she couldn't even take a twenty-minute bath in peace, and Vernon had been terrified because he thought he had been abandoned.

Never rely on the patient's memory to remember what you verbally tell them. Instead, make large signs with simple words and a picture printed in bold magic marker for the most common places you go. When you step out, simply post the sign in plain sight of where the patient normally sits. If Myrleen had hung a sign "IN BATHTUB" with a picture of a woman in a tub and an arrow pointing toward the bathroom, Vernon would not have called his son. Similar signs, such as "IN GARDEN" with a picture of the garden or "GONE TO STORE," will help the patient not panic.

One caregiver posted a large clock with the hands pointing to the time she would return from the store. She included a note that read, "Back by…"

I find patients who were literate before developing AD usually retain their ability to read and comprehend simple three-word phrases long after they lose their ability to remember what someone verbally tells them. For pictures, you can print them off the internet, cut them out of magazines, or draw them by hand.

Most patients shadow their caregiver because they are bored. AD robs them of their ability to self-direct their free time and do activities that used to give them pleasure. Thus, they rely on their caregiver to fill their day.

Often you can assign tasks that go along with what you are already doing. When doing laundry, have them separate the whites from the colors, or load the washing machine, or separate the forks, spoons and knives as you empty the dishwasher. Until late stage, they can fold towels, socks, and T-shirts. You can always fix whatever mistakes they make. The goal is to keep them busy. Dusting with a Swiffer and vacuuming are simple tasks they can do, and it also makes them feel needed. Feeding junk mail into a paper shredder can keep them busy.

In the yard, patients can mulch, dig up crab grass, deadhead flowers, or water the garden with a hose. Yes, it may take longer doing it together, but the job gets done, and the patient feels useful. Chapter 17 lists activities patients can perform until they become bed-bound.

Constant Negativity

Caregivers often express frustration that their parent or spouse with AD is always negative. They don't want to eat what you prepare, they don't want to wear what you pick out, or they don't want to go to the senior citizens center or to church. In short, the patient turns into a total killjoy. "It's hard to stay positive when he is so negative about everything," one frustrated wife told me. "I've reached the point I don't even want to be around him, let alone try to make him happy." Perhaps these suggestions can help:

First, give the patient choices whenever possible. "Dad, do you want macaroni and cheese or chicken noodle soup for lunch?" "Do you want to wear your blue shirt or your green shirt?" "Which do you want to do first—eat breakfast or take your bath?" Presenting choices can help because it allows the patient some control.

AD has robbed him of so much, and he is frustrated he can't be independent anymore. Consequently, you become the scapegoat to his frustration. But here's a helpful secret: When presented with a choice of two options, most AD patients select the second one. Why? Because it was the last one presented, and they can remember it better. Thus, if you would prefer to fix chicken noodle soup over macaroni and cheese, make soup the second option you offer.

Second, offer choices whenever you can, even in the small decisions. If the patient has to take her shower now and not later, you can say, "Mom, do you want to use the shampoo that smells like lilacs or the one that smells like coconuts?" Then let her smell each bottle and decide. It can even be as simple as, "Do you want to use this blue towel or the fluffy green one?" By distracting Mom with choices, she may not think to protest taking the shower. AD patients can only concentrate on one thing at a time, so peppering them with small decisions will distract them from their negativity.

Third, pick your battles. If your mother refuses to get out of her bathrobe to go to the doctor's office, simply take her in her bathrobe and tell the doctor she refused to change into clean clothes. The doctor will understand, and it will save you a needless feud over something not worth fussing over.

Fourth, remind yourself you can't make her happy. Yes, you can provide a pleasant environment and tasty, nutritious food. You can ensure she gets adequate sleep and good medical care. You can try to distract her when she is grumpy or bored, but if she persists in always seeing the glass as three-fourths empty, it is out of your control. Release yourself from the burden of thinking you have to make her happy. Happiness is a mindset, and much of her unhappiness stems from AD robbing her of her independence and ability to do the things she used to do.

Fifth, ask the doctor if the patient might be depressed. While anti-depressants can be tricky with Alzheimer's patients, sometimes they can make a meaningful difference. If the patient is moping around not interested in anything, it's possible they are clinically depressed.

Bed Wetting
Sue Bell

Most Alzheimer's patients will occasionally wet the bed, even when wearing disposable diapers. This is especially true in the later stages when the patient loses bladder control or no longer registers the need to go to the bathroom.

My husband had sensitive skin, so it was important to keep him dry. Changing an entire bed in the middle of the night quickly grew tiresome. Fortunately, I developed a timesaving method to keep Ray dry at night without having to strip and re-make the entire bed. Here is my solution:

Purchase the proper supplies:

1. A cloth, fitted, waterproof mattress cover
2. Several sets of sheets (fitted and flat)
3. Disposable or non-disposable pads

Disposable pads are available at drug stores, while non-disposable, washable pads are found at medical supply stores. The non-disposable pads come in different sizes, but I found the 20-by-30-inch size was sufficient. Non-disposable pads are cheaper, but they must be laundered and so will increase your workload. (Tip: The non-disposable pads will last longer and stay more flexible if you let them air dry after washing rather than using the dryer.)

Make the bed in layers:

- First, place a cloth, waterproof mattress cover on top of the regular mattress. The clear plastic mattress covers are not advised because they are slippery, and patients can slide off the bed and get injured.
- Second, place a fitted sheet on top of the mattress cover.
- Third, place a 20-by-30-inch waterproof pad on top of the fitted sheet in the middle of the bed.

- Next, place a second fitted sheet on top of the waterproof pad.
- Finally, place a second 20-by-30-inch waterproof pad on top of the second fitted sheet. Then add your top sheet, blankets, and bedspread as usual. Below is a diagram of a properly made bed:

<u>Bed-Layering Procedure</u>

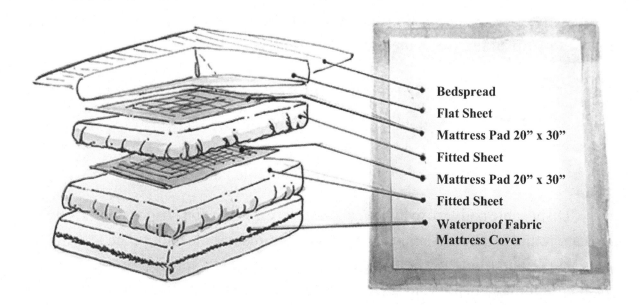

Bedspread

Flat Sheet

Mattress Pad 20" x 30"

Fitted Sheet

Mattress Pad 20" x 30"

Fitted Sheet

Waterproof Fabric
Mattress Cover

With this foolproof method, if Ray had an accident at night because his disposable underwear didn't hold, I merely had to change his underwear and remove the top waterproof pad and the top fitted sheet if it was wet. The bottom waterproof pad and fitted sheet held until morning. This setup saved me a lot of time and hassle since I didn't have to do a complete bed change in the middle of the night. I started a small wash cycle with the wet sheet and washable pad immediately so there would be no unappealing smell of urine in the house. Using this system, I could get Ray back into a dry bed—and be back to bed myself—in less than five minutes.

Rolling Out of Bed

During the later stages of AD, patients frequently roll out of bed, which can result in fractures and injuries. There are several ways to keep patients safe:

- Use a hospital bed with railings.
- If they are still limber, put their mattress on the floor.
- Attach bed rails to the bed.
- Slide a piece of furniture, such as a chest of drawers, against the bed and have the other side of the bed against the wall.
- Place a twin mattress on the floor next to the bed. That way, if your patient rolls off, they will have a soft landing.

Overreacting

When AD patients feel threatened, overwhelmed, or if they fear having their cognitive deficits exposed (such as at a doctor's appointment or large family gathering where they cannot answer all the questions thrown at them), they may overreact, scream, throw things, refuse to get out of the car, bite, hit, or become combative. Doctors refer to these outbursts as "catastrophic reactions."

Baths and getting ready to go out are frequent triggers. This is one of the most frustrating aspects of caretaking. You are in a hurry to get Mom bathed, dressed, and out the door for her doctor's appointment, but she is dawdling and resisting you at every turn. As a physician, I've had dozens of exasperated caregivers call the office to cancel appointments at the last minute because they could not get their loved one to cooperate. So what do you do?

First, look for the cause of the patient's obstinacy. Are they dreading the doctor's visit? If so, gentle assurance can help. Hold her hand and say, "I'll be right next to you, Mom. I won't let anybody harm you." Assess if they are tired, hungry, or in pain. Are they feeling overwhelmed by the complexity of the task you are asking of them? Are they feeling patronized or demeaned?

Second, don't mention the task that upsets them until they calm down. Distract them by singing their favorite song with a cheerful voice or pointing to the birds at the feeder.

Third, break down the complex task into small, unintimidating steps. With a calm voice say, "Let's walk to the bathroom," rather than, "Go take a bath." Once she is in the bathroom say, "I love the smell of this lavender bubble bath, don't you? Let's pour some in the warm water I've already got in the tub." Then, "Let's unbutton this dirty, old bathrobe so I can wash it," and so on, until the task is done.

Fourth, use distraction. Resume singing her favorite hymn while undressing her to minimize her embarrassment about being naked.

Fifth, if she won't cooperate, simply bring her to the doctor's office in her bathrobe and slippers. Explain to the nurse and doctor that you couldn't get her to cooperate with changing into clean clothes. Trust me, the doctor will understand and would rather have the patient show up in her bathrobe than not at all. As a doctor, I have treated many patients in their bathrobes.

Sixth, never yell at the patient. While you might yell at your teenaged son if he neglects to drag the garbage bin to the street after being reminded several times, yelling at an AD patient never brings about cooperation. It only makes her agitated, and things may escalate into a catastrophic reaction.

Agitated Alzheimer's patients are some of the most stubborn and dangerous patients with whom I have worked. You cannot reason with them, and they are too big to force into doing what you want. In power struggles, the caregiver almost always loses and comes out frustrated and mentally exhausted. If you reach the point you want to yell at your patient, take a five-minute break. Take slow, deep, cleansing breaths, roll your neck, and clear your mind by picturing yourself on the beach listening to waves and seagulls. Only when you have calmed down and feel more in control of your emotions should you try again. This time, avoid using the word "bath" altogether. Sometimes just using different words such as "nice, warm wash cloth" instead of "bath" can solicit cooperation.

If the patient still insists she doesn't want to do something, acknowledge her feelings but progress to the next step anyway. "I know you don't want to take a bath, Mom. It's a lot of work for both of us, isn't it? Let's just walk to the bathroom and clean up with a washcloth instead." Scoop the patient's legs into a standing position and distract her while you lead her to the bathroom by talking about the weather, how pretty the roses are, how much you love chocolate chip cookies—anything to get her mind off the task she doesn't want to do. Sing "Row, Row, Row Your Boat" or a familiar childhood song to distract the patient.

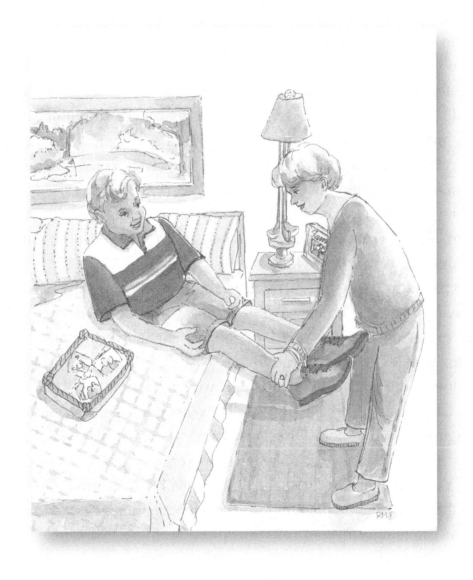

Remember, distraction is your best friend. If she still resists, let it go for ten minutes, then try again by breaking the task into smaller steps. If she still won't cooperate, forget the bath altogether and clean her with a washcloth as best you can. Sometimes you have to lose the power struggle for the sake of harmony. Pick your battles.

"I Want to Go Home"

At some point, most patients will insist they "want to go home," even if they have lived in their current house for sixty years. What do they mean by this? Do they want to go to the home of their childhood? Do they want to go back to a time when they felt comfortable and happy? Are they talking about their heavenly home? Or do they have an unmet need they simply cannot communicate.

They may feel afraid or powerless with all the changes that are occurring. Perhaps they no longer recognize their house and want to return to a place that feels safe, comfortable, and familiar from fifty years ago.

Telling the patient that he *is* home doesn't necessarily help. It often only agitates him. Why? Because in his mind, he is not in the place he remembers as home, and thus, you are lying to him.

Your patient is living in a different reality now. I personally cannot imagine how frightening it would be to wake up in the world of Alzheimer's disease, a world that exists only in the mind of the patient, a world where he doesn't recognize his own home or his own wife.

Ask him to tell you about the home he wants to return to. "What did you like most about that house?" "Who lived there?" "What made it a special place?" Your goal is to figure out what "home" means to him. Often, old pictures of a childhood home or a picture with siblings from when they were teenagers will help bring back a memory. You can then say, "It sounds like a lovely home, Dad. No wonder you want to go there. We should plan to go for a visit sometime. How about we go get a snack now. I'm hungry."

Validate his feelings about what home means, and don't dismiss his desire to go back, but then distract him.

Ray would sometimes wake up around 2:00 a.m. and begin to pack a suitcase, saying, "I'm going home." We were in the home we had built and lived in for forty years. I would try to reason with him, but he kept packing. He would generally say, "I'll come back tomorrow, but I have to go home tonight." At first, I tried telling him he was home. Big mistake! When that didn't work, I would try to delay him by using distraction until he forgot about his plans to leave. I would say things like: "It's dark outside. You can't see well enough to drive safely at night. Let's go home in the morning after you've had a good night of sleep." Or, "I need to wash and iron those shirts before you pack them." My goal was simply to delay and distract him.

What usually worked best was to say, "Let's go eat a cookie and milk so you won't be hungry when you go." As we sat at the kitchen table eating his favorite cookie and drinking hot chocolate, I would try to create a place that felt safe and caring. I would serve the hot chocolate in his favorite mug, and we would sit at the familiar kitchen table where I served every meal. I would speak in a calm and reassuring voice and comment on how delicious the cookies and cocoa were. After a while, when he had calmed down and had clearly forgotten about leaving, I would suggest we go back to bed. This always worked.

Once again, distraction is your best friend!

~ FYI: People who have placed a loved one in a nursing home often express guilt when they cannot keep their loved one at home, especially when the patient constantly expresses a desire to "go home." Both my husband and mother stayed at home until the day they died, yet even so, both talked about wanting to "go home." ~

Agitation

Some patients with moderate to late stage AD have moments of extreme agitation that manifests itself with moaning, pacing, and handwringing for no apparent reason. It is often worse after dusk and can be triggered by seemingly trivial things. Calming an agitated patient can be exhausting. Here are a few things to try:

- Give the patient a security object such as a stuffed toy. Just as a toddler can find comfort in a beloved stuffed animal, some later stage AD patients find comfort when sleeping with one as well. Give the stuffed animal a name and talk to it lovingly.

- If you have a gentle cat or dog, ask the patient to give the pet some love. Stroking a pet is calming.

- Play a CD of favorite hymns or songs and sing along. Music calms many patients.

- If it is not too dark, go for a short walk with the patient. This will dissipate some of the excess adrenalin. Point out the flowers, squirrels or anything that can distract the patient.

- Try doing a gentle hand or foot massage using a pleasant-smelling lotion. Maintain a calm, soothing voice.

- Put on their favorite movie.

Obsessing about People or Pets that Are Dead

AD patients frequently get it in their head that a dead family member or pet is lost or missing. I know of patients who roamed the streets in the middle of the night looking for a cat that had died years earlier. AD patients have gotten lost roaming the woods behind their houses while searching for a long-dead dog. If informed the pet or family member died two years earlier, they may become agitated. They won't believe you, or if they do, they won't remember what you said ten minutes from now. Plus, in their mind, the beloved pet or sister is still alive.

So how do you deal with an AD patient who insists a dead cat is lost and needs rescuing?

- Jim B. got his grandmother to calm down and go to bed by promising he would make sure the missing cat was okay. As his wife put Granny to bed, she reassured her, "Jim will take care of Fluffy." Jim went through the motions of finding a flashlight, putting on his winter coat, and going outside for several minutes in a feigned search for the missing cat. By morning, his grandmother had forgotten all about the dead cat—at least for awhile.

- Sometimes a lighthearted comment works. "Dad is on vacation with Jesus," or "I'll have to give St. Peter a call and find out how Rover is doing."

What I find works best is to share fond memories about the dead pet or loved one. Reminisce about their endearing qualities. Comments such as, "Fluffy was such a nice kitty, wasn't she? I loved her loud purr." Ask your loved one what she most remembers about the beloved pet (or person). Share how much you loved the cedar chest your father made for a wedding gift, or how much you enjoyed the family vacation to the Grand Canyon.

~ Share treasured memories about the dead person or pet to distract the patient until you can change the subject. You need not mention that the beloved pet or relative is dead: It will only upset them. ~

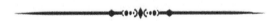

Unwanted Sexual Behavior

Dr. Sally Burbank

Sometimes patients will touch or fondle their privates when they have a wet pull-up or have to go to the bathroom, so don't assume all touching in the private area is sexual. If you see the patient self-touching, say, "Let's take you to the bathroom, Dad."

Never shame the patient, even if he is fondling his genitals. He no longer knows this is inappropriate in public. Instead, find something else to occupy his time that uses his hands—stroking the cat, folding laundry, dusting with a Swiffer, feeding paper into a paper shredder, playing with a Rubik's cube.

If the patient makes unwelcomed sexual advances, use humor and distraction. Wave your index finger and say, "Now, now, Mr. Jones. No hanky-panky with me. You wouldn't want me to have a heart attack, would you?" or, "Let's find something better to do with those hands of yours, shall we?" or, "I bet you were a real lady's man in your prime, weren't you. Too bad I'm a married woman."

When in public, keep printed cards handy that say, "He has severe Alzheimer's and doesn't know what he is doing. Please forgive his inappropriate behavior." Be ready to hand one to whoever the patient offends, smile, apologize, then quickly usher your loved one away.

If inappropriate sexual behavior becomes a common problem, purchase an activity apron from Amazon, also known as a "busy apron." This gives him something to do with his hands.

If you are married but no longer want to be sexual with your husband—because you feel more like his nurse than his lover—a back rub, hug, snuggle, or hand holding can often meet the patient's need for touch and affection. You can say, "I don't have the energy for that tonight, but I'd love to give you a hug and hold your hand.

Is it wrong for a married couple to have sex if one of them is demented? Not if the experience is enjoyable, or at least tolerable, to both. Your wife may not know who you are anymore, but she may still crave the cuddling and affection she was accustomed to getting throughout your marriage. Just because a partner isn't cognitively sharp doesn't mean his or her need for love has abated, and for some AD patients, the sex drive is still strong.

If you as the caregiver are sexually turned off because of the radical changes AD has caused in your relationship, are you obligated to have relations anyway? When the patient doesn't know who you are anymore, it can feel wrong—like you're having sex with a stranger.

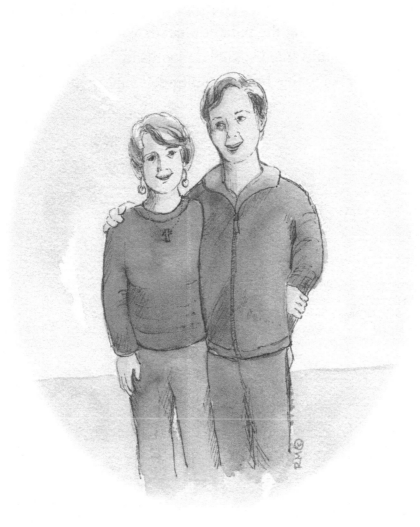

Many wives struggle with guilt over this issue. They feel like it is their "marital duty" to have sex with their husband if he wants it, but they find the experience distasteful or somehow degrading. One wife tearfully confessed to me, "I don't feel like his cherished wife when he doesn't even know who I am anymore. I don't think he would care if it were me or the cleaning lady. I dread sex and look for excuses to get out of it. Then I feel guilty because he still seems to enjoy it. It's not his fault he has Alzheimer's, and I promised to love him 'in sickness and in health.' Am I a terrible wife for declining his sexual desires?"

Feelings like these can and should be discussed with a trusted friend, support group, pastor, or counselor. Often, cuddling, hugging, holding hands and simple gestures of affection will meet the patient's needs without intercourse, or you can distract the patient from unwanted sexual demands by bringing up another subject, asking a question, or showing him something. Once again, distraction is your friend!

CHAPTER 21

ISN'T LYING WRONG?
Dr. Sally Burbank

Most of us have had it drummed into our heads since we were toddlers that lying is wrong and even sinful. So what do you do as a caregiver when telling your loved one the truth may cause unnecessary anxiety or grief?

"I need to be honest with Mother," you tell yourself, but when you try to set the facts straight, you are rewarded with an agitated patient who doesn't believe you anyway. In her mind, what you are telling her is the lie!

Even worse, your truthful words may trigger an emotional melt down. ("My son Tony died? When?") In fact, Tony died three years ago, and the patient even attended the funeral, but now she is reacting as though she is hearing the news for the first time. You reminded her several times before that Tony died in a car crash, but in her mind, Tony is still very much alive. Every time you tell her Tony is dead, she plunges back into shock and grief because, in her world, this is the first time she is hearing the news. You've just made her re-live the worst day of her life all over again. Why do this? What is gained by your honesty, especially when she won't remember it in an hour anyway?

In this case, blunt honesty is not the best thing. A better response would be to make a kind comment about Tony: "Tony's barbecued ribs were so tender, they fell off the bone." This isn't lying, and more importantly, it doesn't fling your mother off an emotional cliff.

Attempts to pull your loved one back into the world of reality is pointless and will only agitate her. It is far kinder to enter her world and ask, "What do you remember about your home? What made it so special?" By entering her world, you allow her to reminisce about a home that made her feel happy and secure.

I like to tell caregivers that if they have a choice between blunt honesty or

---

kindness, kindness wins out every time. The Bible says the greatest commandment is love—to love God and to love others. Instead of cramming honesty down Dad's throat in a futile attempt to re-orient him, go into his world and try to make it better by asking questions or providing reassurances.

Most of us wouldn't be cruel enough to tell a three-year-old shopping with her mother on Christmas Eve that Santa Claus is a myth and that her parents have lied to her. Why? Because in that child's world, Santa Claus does exist. To tell her otherwise would needlessly traumatize her.

There are, of course, times when the caregiver is forced to be honest and must try to gently re-direct the patient into reality. When Sally's father woke up from a vivid dream in the middle of a freezing winter night convinced he had to go outside to gather hay bales to stack them in the barn before it rained, Sally's mother had no choice but to point at the two feet of snow and sub-zero temperature on the thermometer and remind him that haying is not done in the middle of the winter. "It was just a vivid dream," she reassured him. She then softened her words by saying, "I've had dreams that seemed real, too." This allowed my father to save face. Mom had to speak the truth, or my father would have trudged out in the snow looking for hay bales in the middle of February! She spoke the truth with love and kindness.

In short, before correcting an AD patient, ask yourself these questions:

- Does it really matter?
- Will telling the truth needlessly agitate her?
- Will she remember what I tell her an hour from now?
- Would not telling her the truth lead to harm in some way?
- Would she be better off if I go along with her sense of reality?

Remember, the goal as a caregiver is to keep your loved one calm and safe. If correcting misinformation hinders this goal, let it go.

~ Love and kindness trump blunt honesty. ~

CHAPTER 22

◆‹••›◗◆◖‹••›◆

WHERE *IS* HE?
Sue Bell

My husband disappeared three times. Three nerve-racking, nail-biting, where-is-he??? times!

The first time Ray left home, I was still working, and he had retired. He left home that morning to play golf at a familiar golf course about twenty-two miles away. When I came home from work, he wasn't there. This was unusual, as he always called home if he was going to be late. Even though cell phones were common in 2004, Ray didn't own one.

I called every place I could think of where he frequented during the day, but no one had seen him.

As night came and there was still no word, I called the police. They insisted I file a missing person report. This was upsetting for many reasons: It meant admitting something bad had happened, such as an accident or medical problem. I never considered he was lost due to a memory issue, since he had played at that golf course dozens of times. I knew his memory wasn't good, (he had trouble with names, dates, and details—problems many people face as they age), but I never suspected he had Alzheimer's disease.

The missing person report was sent out, along with a picture, to every police station. Our friends and family members began searching for him. At this point, we assumed he'd gotten in an accident or had experienced a fatal heart attack. The police enlisted the assistance of other government agencies, like school bus drivers.

The day after the All-Points Bulletin was sent out, a police officer in a town about fifty miles away called to say that prior to the APB, he had run the car tags when my husband stopped him, said he was lost, and asked for directions. He had even offered the officer a soda after getting the information. The officer described my husband as very polite, and he said everything seemed normal.

We realized now we had to expand our search to outside our county. The police informed the bank to watch his credit cards—they knew he would eventually need to purchase food, gas, or lodging. Though it was a relief to know he had not had an accident or heart attack, I now had new worries to face: Why had he left? Why hadn't he called? Where was he? Was he okay?

Two harrowing days after my husband left home, a call came from a police department in Ellisville, Mississippi. The police had found him. Ray had gone into a gas station to buy a soda. When he asked the clerk if she had seen his wife, she noticed something strange about his behavior. She said he reminded her of her grandfather who had Alzheimer's disease.

A local police officer happened to come in, and the clerk asked the officer to check on him. When the officer talked to him, Ray said he was waiting on his wife. "I'm supposed to meet her here," he insisted, though he didn't know where "here" was, the day of the week, his phone number, or his address.

The officer ran his tags and the APB alert came up. They called our local police department, who notified me Ray had been found eight hours from our home. He had no clue where he was or how long he'd been gone, and he couldn't remember what he had done during the three days.

We looked for clues once he got home. He had no money in his wallet, and there was a red baseball cap in his truck along with a bag of oranges. But he always kept money in his wallet, he never wore red, and he didn't like oranges: Someone else must have ridden in the truck! Had he picked up a hitchhiker along the way? I said, "Ray you wouldn't pick up a hitchhiker, would you?" He replied, "I might, if I could help him."

He never regained memory of those three days. When I described what had happened, he said, "Why would I do something like that?" He couldn't believe the event had even happened. To prove it, I showed him the flier we had made of him while he was missing.

Prior to this incident, if you had told me my husband would leave home for three days, travel eight hours away without even realizing it, and would later be diagnosed with dementia: I would never have believed you. Ray was an educated, intelligent, practical, and extremely cautious man. He had been a teacher, coach, principal, insurance agent, and mayor of our town. It was a shock to realize he didn't simply suffer from a bad memory: he had something far more devastating.

The second time Ray went missing, we were at my mom's house eating lunch and visiting with family members. The next thing we knew, Ray was missing. He had taken the keys off the kitchen counter, hopped in the car and driven off. We had no idea where he was, so we all immediately took off looking for him. When we found him, he was aimlessly driving around town. Luckily, we were able to pull him over and get him out of the car.

The third time, I ran in to pay a bill at our local insurance office, and I left Ray asleep in the car for the few minutes it would take. When I returned to the car, he was gone. We eventually found him at a local McDonalds standing in line to place an order.

IDENTIFICATION—A MUST!
Dr. Sally Burbank and Sue Bell

Once your loved one has been diagnosed with AD and you are watching out for him on a regular basis, you may think you don't have to worry about him getting lost. Wrong! In the time it takes you to shower, run to the store for milk, or merely go to the bathroom, the patient can wander off. Therefore, it is essential that _all_ AD patients carry identification on them at _all_ times. That way, someone can reach you if the patient becomes lost.

Life Alert devices, where the patient can push a button if they are lost, are not reliable with AD patients—they often don't remember to push the button!

Reports about Alzheimer's patients who have gone missing is upsetting. Fortunately, there are now many things you can do to help them live safely.

Patients are most likely to wander off after they have moved from their home into a son or daughter's house, or into an assisted living or nursing home facility. They are usually intent upon returning to their old house, often clueless that it may be miles away or even sold. Others wander off looking for the caregiver if the caregiver gets out of their sight. Be sure the patient always has a bracelet stating he has dementia. Put his first name, your name, address, and cell phone number on the bracelet.

Never rely on the patient's ability to remember what you tell him: he won't. When he realizes he is alone, he may panic and wander off to look for you. Instead, if your loved one can still read and comprehend simple words, write a note in big magic marker letters and tape it to the door. Keep it simple, such as, "Gone to grocery store. Be back soon. Stay in house." Or, "In the garden." If the patient can comprehend the note, they won't panic.

Every morning, tuck a fully-charged (and turned on!) cell phone with a "Find iPhone" or "Life 360" app into the patient's pocket or into a fanny pack around their waist. That way, in addition to being able to call the patient directly, (if they're still able to comprehend and answer it), you will be able to locate the patient by locating the phone. Be sure to re-charge the battery every night. Tape your phone number in large print on the back of the phone. Also, enter your name and number into the phone's contact list and have the patient practice calling you. Never leave the cell phone turned off in an effort to avoid using up the charge: the tracker device won't work if the phone is turned off. Plus, many AD patients, when addled, won't remember how to turn the phone on or how to use it. They may try to call you with the phone turned off and get frustrated. They may even throw the phone away thinking it is broken.

Practice locating the patient's cellphone using the "Find iPhone" or "Life 360" phone app ahead of time, so you won't have to scramble learning how to do it during a crisis. Also, have your patient practice taking the phone out of their pocket and answering it when it rings.

Many lives have been saved because of this simple phone app. If you can't figure out how to install or operate it, ask a clerk at your cell phone vendor to install it, or get one of your kids or grandkids to help you.

There are also GPS locating systems that can be worn as a shoe insert or a bracelet. These will only be effective, however, if they remain charged. If your loved one is tempted to grab the car keys and go for a drive, a GPS locator placed discretely in the car would allow you to locate where the patient has gone.

A non-profit organization called Project Lifesaver International provides GPS bracelets to those with AD and other mental handicaps. So far, over 2,000 lost individuals have been located thanks to these bracelets. Their website is www.projectlifesaver.org.

Another option is to purchase a Safe Return bracelet from the Alzheimer's Association. For $55 plus shipping, you will receive a bracelet with your patient's first name, ID number, and a toll-free phone number to call 24/7. If your loved one is lost, anyone who sees the bracelet can call the number and be put in touch with the person whose information has been entered into the Alzheimer's Association's data bank. The bracelet also alerts the rescuer that your loved one is memory-challenged. Unlike cheaper Medic Alert bracelets that are easy for the patient to take off, these bracelets are double-clasped, so the patient cannot remove them. Remind the patient daily that if he ever gets lost, he can show someone his bracelet. The annual renewal fee is $35 (in 2018). Caregiver bracelets are also available, which alert others that if you, the caregiver, become incapacitated, you have a loved one with Alzheimer's at home who needs immediate attention.

If a loved one goes missing, the caregiver can call Safe Return, and they will FAX a photo and description of the patient to the appropriate police departments. Safe Return will already have a photo of your loved one in their data bank.

The Safe Return program started in 1993, and since then, more than 5,000 lost patients have been reunited with their caregivers. To obtain the bracelet and learn more about recommended steps you can take to protect your loved one, call the Alzheimer's Association at (800) 272-3900, or to just order the bracelets, call (888) 572-8566, or visit their website at: alz.org

If your loved one goes missing, notify the police immediately. The local news recently reported on a man with Alzheimer's disease who was working in the yard with his wife when she suddenly noticed he had wandered off. She called the police, and since he normally could walk only a block or two, she wasn't too worried. Amazingly, the police found him a full two miles from the house. He didn't know his name or address, but he insisted he was going to buy his wife flowers for Mother's Day, which was the next day. Apparently, he had given her flowers every year since their first child was born, and he was determined to go to a local florist to purchase them. The policeman took him to buy the flowers and even helped pay for them, since the patient didn't have enough money to cover the cost. Upon his safe return, the wife said, "The heart never forgets."

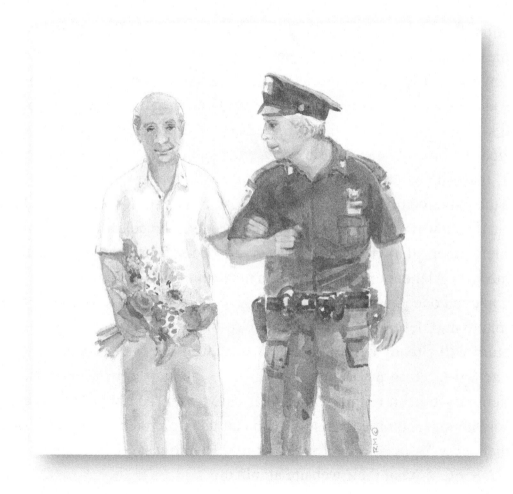

Unfortunately, another news story didn't end so well. An elderly man went missing from his home early one morning in the dead of winter. He was found the next day, frozen to death. He had gotten out of the house without his caregiver's knowledge and wasn't found until it was too late.

Stop by the homes of your neighbors who live within a mile or so of your home and get to know them. Leave a page with a picture of your loved one and an explanation that he has AD and might wander from home and get lost. Include a picture of your house. With the picture, provide the patient's name and your contact information. Ask the neighbors to call you if they ever see him walking alone. The information could be put in a discrete envelope and handed to the neighbor as "Important information I'd like you to keep." Perhaps your loved one could offer each neighbor a homemade cookie as an excuse for the visit.

I know of one case where a flyer such as this saved a patient's life. While her caregiver slept, an elderly woman with AD woke in the middle of the night convinced her cat, who had died two years earlier, was outside freezing to death. Garbed in just a nightgown and slippers, she ventured out into the sub-zero night air, hollering the name of her cat. Like many AD patients, she seemed clueless that she was inappropriately attired for below-freezing temperatures.

Thankfully, a neighbor saw the patient and remembered the flyer she had received months earlier alerting her to call if she ever saw the woman alone. The neighbor—a nurse—was driving home after her evening shift. She stopped to inquire, and when informed of the missing cat, offered to help as a way to get the woman into her warm car. She told the patient they would find the cat faster driving in the car. She then drove home, located the flyer, and called the caregiver. The patient was returned home safe and sound before she froze to death.

Alzheimer's patients can be very trusting. Thankfully, this neighbor had good intentions. Ironically, AD patients will sometimes refuse to get into the car of the police officer who locates them because they are afraid. Thankfully, most cops are trained in dealing with AD and use a calm voice and gentle demeanor.

~ Personal identification is a must. No excuses. Get it done! ~

CHAPTER 23

————◆————

VIOLENT AND AGITATED PATIENTS
Dr. Sally Burbank

As the disease progresses into the moderately severe stage, close to 50 percent of patients display extreme agitation, anger, or irrational rage. In fact, the number one reason caregivers give for eventually resorting to using a nursing home is because their patient becomes unmanageable, aggressive, or so emotionally unpredictable the caregiver no longer feels safe. Fortunately, only 5-10 percent of patients become physically violent. Be aware, however, that the way caregivers and others respond to the patient can unwittingly trigger unwanted behavior. It is important to learn how to avoid aggravating and inciting the patient.

What should I expect?

Early Stage: Patients may be irritable, argumentative, and unreasonable. When tired or over-stimulated, they may become agitated and pace the floor. With rest, they usually return to their baseline personality. Unfortunately, those who were stubborn and demanding before AD tend to become more so as the disease progresses. Those who were naturally sweet tend to stay that way—unless they feel threatened or challenged.

Moderate Stage: Episodes of irritability and uncooperativeness become more frequent. Getting the patient to take a bath, eat healthy food, or wear clean clothing can become a huge ordeal. The simplest request can turn into a power struggle. They misplace things and forget where they stashed them. They spend their money, but then accuse family members of stealing it, because they don't remember spending it. Accusations of stealing are extremely upsetting to family members. "How can Mom think I'd steal from her?" one tearful daughter asked.

Loud music, repetitive noises, boisterous conversations, rowdy laughter, disrespectful teenagers, shrieking children, or angry arguments may set them off. Patients get flustered and overwhelmed when they don't recognize people who seem to know them, or when they can't follow the gist of a conversation. In frustration, they may curse, (even if they never cursed in pre-AD days), lose their temper, or throw things at the person annoying them. Often the trigger seems trivial. When agitated, they may pace, tear paper, or perform other senseless repetitive actions. If you badger them to eat, or if you serve something they don't want, they may throw food at you or onto the floor. In short, their behavior becomes impulsive and reactionary.

Moderately Severe Stage: In this stage, 5-10 percent of patients become violent and may assault people when agitated. One of my patients had to put her mother in a nursing home after her mother chased the twelve-year-old grandchild around the house with a butcher knife. The poor girl locked herself in the bathroom until her mother returned home and rescued her from Grandma.

Another patient heaved his knee into his physical therapist's crotch when the therapist harangued him to do one more set of knee exercises. "Nothing wrong with that knee," the patient hissed at the poor therapist, who was bent over double in pain. "Want me to show you how well my other knee works?" he threatened.

Late Stage: Patients may hallucinate, become paranoid, see and hear things, or insist a creak in the house means a thief has broken in. One AD patient nearly clobbered his wife with a baseball bat when he heard her get up in the night to go to the bathroom. He no longer recognized her as his wife and thought she was an intruder.

Patients may have trouble differentiating between dreams and reality. One patient used to wake up screaming after a recurring nightmare in which he was cornered by a pack of snarling wolves. His wife would spend the next thirty minutes trying to convince him it was all a dream.

When distressed, patients may bite, throw things, say cruel words, or curse. Some AD patients will make inappropriate sexual advances on nurses, and if unmonitored, get hooked on the Playboy channel. A patient of mine was embarrassed when all the nurses she hired to look after her father complained he made lewd sexual comments and tried to grope them. Most refused to come back, and my patient didn't blame them!

In summary, as Alzheimer's progresses, some patients lose all inhibition over their thoughts, behavior, sexual urges, and words. But on a positive note, this violent, hateful stage usually doesn't last for more than a year. As the disease advances, the patient will become mute and far less aggressive.

Why do they become violent?

The hippocampus, frontal lobe, and pre-frontal cortex of the brain control emotional response, planning, rational thought, and inhibition of inappropriate words or behaviors. These areas of the brain act as the "brake" on impulsivity. Unfortunately, Alzheimer's disease preferentially attacks and destroys brain cells in these areas. This means the patient loses the ability to think before he speaks or reacts.

What triggers patients to act out?

- **Overstimulation**—especially late in the day. Too many appointments and long interactions with people they don't remember can quickly exhaust the patient and further erode self-control. Patients are especially irritated by heated political debates, arguments, and shouting. When they cannot keep up with the conversation around them, they show their frustration by lashing out verbally or physically.

- **Change in living quarters**—such as moving in with a child or into a nursing home or assisted living facility. Hospital admissions, with the constant stream of nurses, doctors, therapists, and visitors, are especially confusing to the patient. Also, infection, anesthesia, low oxygen levels, and the inability to understand what is happening around them—all contribute to the sundowning behavior notoriously seen during the hospital's graveyard shift.

- **Bossy caregivers**—like nurses or other caregivers who try to make the patient take a bath, eat lunch, change clothes, do physical therapy, etc., against their will. Though dependent on others to care for them, AD patients don't like being bossed around, so give them a choice whenever possible.

- **Frustration**—such as when they can't find something they've squirreled away or can't do something they used to do. Frustration builds when they can no longer express what they need because they cannot pull up the right words to communicate.

- **Arguing or insisting the patient is wrong**—because in the patient's mind, the caregiver is wrong. The more the caregiver insists, "Your brother John died last year. Don't you remember?", the more agitated the patient becomes. The more you insist Mom probably misplaced her checkbook, the more likely she will claim you stole it.

- **Vision and hearing loss**—because not being able to see is disorienting, and not being able to hear, understand, and follow a conversation is frustrating.

- **Pain**—such as the chronic pain from an arthritic hip or a bad back.

- **Fatigue**—such as when a patient has a delayed bedtime or misses an afternoon nap. Patients are usually at their best first thing in the morning after breakfast. They are most likely to become ornery or unreasonable in the late afternoon or early evening.

- **Sensing anger, impatience, or frustration in those around them**—such as when family members argue or act put-out that the patient doesn't remember what he was told five minutes ago.

- **Threats to take away the patient's autonomy**—such as revoking driving privileges, money management, or the right to live in one's own home. When confronted with bounced checks or the ability to pay utility bills on time, they may become incensed and insist they are perfectly capable of taking care of themselves.

———

These are the hardest conversations, because the patient will flatly deny they can't drive safely, live alone, or handle money. When you give examples to demonstrate their inabilities, they may accuse you of wanting to steal their money or get rid of them. They accuse doctors of being "quacks" and claim you don't care about them. Patients will play the guilt card, because it is the only card they have left! They may insist you never come to see them, even if you were there yesterday. Why? Because they don't remember. They have lost the ability to judge time, so, feeling abandoned, they act out.

- **Medications.** Unfortunately, I have seen Aricept and drugs commonly used to treat Alzheimer's disease cause personality changes and aggression in some patients. Discuss the patient's meds with your doctor.

Tips for Reducing Aggressive Behavior

- **Offer the hand of grace.** Remember that the awful behavior and hateful words are due to a brain disease. The patient is not intentionally being cruel or difficult.

- **Diffuse tension by changing the subject.** If your ninety-year-old father with AD insists his mother is still alive, don't correct him. Instead, change the subject by saying something nice about his mother: "Granny made the best beef stew," or, "Your mother sure grew pretty roses." Deflect what they say rather than focus on the inaccuracy. Teach everyone who has contact with the patient to expect questions or comments to be repeated. Do not respond, "Don't you remember? I answered that two minutes ago." Instead, repeat your answer and then try to distract the patient.

- **Use distraction.** Just as fussy toddlers can be easily distracted, so can most AD patients. If a particular topic of conversation upsets them, drop it and ask a question about a safe topic, such as their childhood friends or school days. Ask about their first kiss, their first car, or their favorite and least favorite flavors of ice cream. Play some of the patient's favorite music from when they were in their teens and twenties.

- **Avoid overstimulation.** Look to see if the patient is over-stimulated (too much noise, too many people), tired (no afternoon nap), hungry, or feeling threatened.

- **Calm their fears.** If the patient feels afraid, they may react like a caged wild animal. The threat doesn't have to be real. If the patient perceives they are in danger, they will act as if they are.

- **Never argue with the patient.** You will never win. The patient can no longer rationalize, and she won't remember what you say. If you must tell her she can't drive or live alone anymore, don't dwell on the patient's failings. Instead, focus on your love for the patient. Say things like, "I love you too much to risk you getting hurt in a car accident." Or try, "You can't help it that you have Alzheimer's disease. I will make sure you get good care and get to the places you need to go." Or say, "I want to take care of your finances, so no one will take advantage of you." As you say these things, hold the patient's hand and look her in the eye. If she gets angry, stay calm and say, "I see this upsets you, so we won't talk about it anymore." Then smile, give her a hug, and say, "I love you, Mom." In short, diffuse anger with love.

- **Acknowledge and validate the patient's feelings and fears.** Say things like, "I understand how this is frightening (or upsetting) for you, but I promise I won't abandon you. I will make sure you get good care." Comfort the patient and speak love in a calm voice.

- **Never raise your voice or shout at the patient, no matter how much they addle you.** Remember, the patient does not have a fully functioning brain, but you do! If you find yourself wanting to yell, give yourself a ten-minute time-out to calm down. If you raise your voice, the patient's emotions may escalate to the point of anger, rage, or even violence. Instead, make noncommittal statements like, "I see you feel strongly about this," or, "I understand what you're saying, Dad." It doesn't mean you agree; it just means you are listening.

• **Educate everyone in the patient's close circle to not argue with or correct misinformation**—especially young people. Teens and children often think they should correct misinformation, but many AD patients view these well-

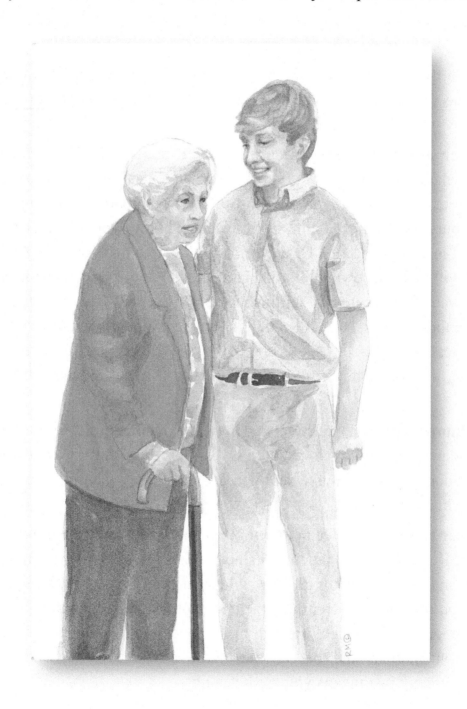

meaning corrections as impertinence. Home health nurses, physical therapists, and sitters all need to be warned not to argue or contradict.

- **Focus on the past and present, not the future.** Alzheimer's patients love to share stories from the past, and they can live in the moment—enjoying colorful flowers, tasty treats, or the antics of a playful puppy. They can enjoy the fun of a birthday party, the giggle of a baby, and favorite old songs. They cannot, however, handle the future, such as remembering upcoming appointments, paying bills on time, or planning and hosting a family Thanksgiving dinner. Focus on what the patient can still do.

- **Avoid complicated directions.** Keep all verbal instructions simple and one-step-at-a-time.

- **Never leave the patient feeling outsmarted or cornered.** Your loved one can no longer rationalize or pull up facts or words easily, so you may be able to outsmart him and win debates, but "winning" comes at a price. The patient may fight in the only way he still can—physically! Avoid needlessly agitating him.

- **Pick your battles.** My father loved card games and won many times throughout his life. As his dementia advanced, however, he could no longer remember that a "run" had to be all from one suit. If we pointed this out, he would slam his cards down and sputter, "Those confounded runs! Now you know what cards I have in my hand!" Since the point of a family game is to have fun, we learned to let it go and say nothing when he mixed a run with both spades and clubs. Dad was allowed to cheat while the rest of us played by the rules. We thought of it as his "handicap" for having dementia. Even with dementia—and his handicap advantage—he still enjoyed skunking us!

- **Apologize even if it wasn't your fault.** If a patient gets really agitated say, "I'm sorry I upset you, Dad." This may defuse the tension.

- **Give patients frequent calm times with no noise.** Turn off the TV and enjoy a cup of herbal tea together. Excess noise addles AD patients.

- **Go for a joy ride.** Car rides soothe AD patients because they can live in the moment. It requires no memory to enjoy a beautiful lilac bush or Monarch butterfly or an interesting Tudor house with turrets.

- **Do the right thing without arguing.** If Mom is ringing up credit cards and forgetting to pay the bills on time, take over the finances. If Dad has no business driving, find a new home for his car. If Mom insists she's fine living alone, but you know she isn't, move her into your house. She may ask daily to move back to her own home, but you can respond with a loving comment like, "I love you too much to risk your safety," or, "I wish you could, but when it comes to safety, it's not up for debate," or, "Getting old isn't for sissies, is it?" Avoid drawn-out discussions and arguments. By tomorrow, your AD patient won't remember the discussions anyhow, and every time you bring it up, it will upset her all over again.

- **Stick to a routine.** Most AD patients do best with a schedule. Most like a big breakfast, a favorite TV show, a ride in the afternoon, and a scoop of ice cream or tasty treat. The more familiar the routine, the calmer the patient.

- **When the patient gets upset or verbally abusive, change the subject.** "Hey, Mom, do you want vanilla ice cream or chocolate pudding for dessert?"

- **Schedule appointments around 9:30-11 a.m.** This is the best time for most Alzheimer's patients. Try to avoid two appointments in one day, as it is often too much. Avoid late afternoon appointments when the doctor may be running behind.

- **Never physically pull on, fight with, or restrain a patient.** You will lose! You may get punched, bit, shoved, or stabbed. When an AD patient feels threatened, he may act like a cornered animal and be surprisingly strong. Instead, leave the room and let him calm down.

- **Try delay tactics.** If a patient insists he is leaving the house or going to do something dangerous, try delaying him. Calmly say, "You can leave, but let's first grab a quick bite so you won't be hungry." Or, "Let's go pack your bags so you'll have everything you need." Then take an inordinate amount of time getting ready, perhaps insisting you need to do a load of wash, so he'll have clean underwear and pants. Then, "How about we get a good night of sleep first, and we can go first thing in the morning?" By morning, he will have forgotten all about leaving. Lock the doors with dead bolts that require a key, and don't let him know where the key is. (See Chapter 28 on Patient Safety for more ideas.)

- **Get all guns out of the house.** No exceptions! If the patient is likely to resist, remove them when the patient is asleep or away. If he notices they are gone, tell him you asked so-and-so to keep them for safekeeping and then change the subject. Many a wife has walked in to see her demented husband cleaning or fiddling with a loaded gun! An AD patient cannot be relied upon to remember all the safety procedures. Even worse, a noise might frighten the patient, and he might shoot someone, thinking the person is an intruder. Don't just hide or lock them up, as AD patients have an uncanny ability to find them. Remember, they love to snoop around.

- **If a patient becomes violent and your safety is at risk, leave the house and call the police.** Have a cell phone with you at all times. Never try to restrain an agitated AD patient by yourself. Sometimes being left alone a few minutes will calm him down better than reasoning with him. Think of it as a time-out.

What about medications for aggressive behavior?

Scientific evidence and government agencies (Medicare) warn that AD patients should NOT use tranquilizers, sleeping pills, or anti-psychotic medications unless the patient is:

- Overtly psychotic (hearing and seeing things/hallucinating)
- A serious danger to themselves or their caretakers
- Agitated and distressed to the point they are pacing, shouting all night, and cannot be soothed using the suggestions listed above.

Studies show that anti-psychotic medications and sleeping pills, such as Ambien, quadruple the risk of hip fractures. Patients on these meds who get up in the night to use the bathroom, or who hear a noise and get up to investigate, are groggy from the drugs and more prone to tripping, falling and fracturing their hips.

Research has also shown there is up to a nine-fold increased risk of stroke in the first four weeks of using anti-psychotic medications (Klijer, 2009), and there is almost a doubling in the risk of mortality (Food and Drug Administration, 2005). In fact, inappropriate prescriptions for sleeping pills and anti-psychotic drugs contribute to 1,800 deaths a year in the United States.

At the annual meeting of the American College of Physicians, Dr. Philip Luber, a professor of psychiatry and associate dean at the University of Texas in San Antonio, recommended that Lexapro (escitalopram) at 5mg starting dose and increasing to 10mg after a month if there is no improvement, or Zoloft (sertraline) at 25-50mg daily can help calm agitated AD patients. Don't assess the effectiveness of the drug for at least a month as these drugs are slow to work. Lexapro and Zoloft must be taken daily and NOT on an "as needed" basis. If these drugs fail, Dr. Luber will next turn to Klonopin (clonazepam) 0.5mg up to twice a day. Only if these medications fail will he turn to anti-psychotics because of the risks mentioned earlier.

If sedation becomes necessary, Risperdal (risperidone) and Seroquel (quetiapine) and Abilify (aripiprazole) have a modest benefit in simmering down the severe agitation and aggression of those with moderate to severe Alzheimer's. Government guidelines suggest not using these anti-psychotics for more than six to twelve weeks, although most violent patients in nursing homes are kept on these drugs until the end stage for the safety of other patients and the staff.

In summary, doctors and caregivers need to carefully assess the risks versus the benefits of using sedating medications or mood-altering medications. Always use the lowest dose that controls the behavior.

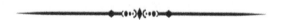

CHAPTER 24

FALLS
Dr. Sally Burbank

Once Alzheimer's disease progresses from the mild to the moderate stage, the risk of falls and fractured hips doubles, compared to non-AD individuals of similar age. Falls start happening around the same time urinary incontinence begins. Why? The part of the brain that controls the bladder lies near the part that controls the legs. By the middle stage, some patients begin to walk with a slow, forward-leaning, shuffling gait, similar to the walk of a Parkinson's patient.

Besides degeneration in the area of the brain that controls leg movement, AD patients may not be able to properly interpret visual clues, such as wet floors, holes in the ground, or uneven pavement. Reflexes are slowed, so the patient's ability to correct or compensate for an uneven surface is delayed. Also, with a shuffling gait, they are more likely to trip over throw rugs and not lift or lower their legs properly on stairs. For that reason, all stairs must have a handrail or railing on each side, or it is an accident waiting to happen.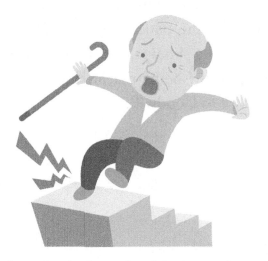

When a patient's balance begins to be impaired, they should start using a rolling walker with a basket and seat when outside the home. Use a quad cane (a cane with four legs at the bottom) around the house.

Remove all throw or scatter rugs, as these are a leading cause of trips and falls.

Holes in the yard or driveway should be filled in with dirt or gravel.

Patients should not walk around the house in slippery socks. Purchase non-slip grip socks if the patient refuses to wear shoes in the house. Sneakers with solid treads and Velcro straps to make them easy to get on and off, are best. These can be purchased online if your local shoe stores don't carry them.

All showers should have grab bars to assist with getting in and out. Grab bars at the commode also reduce the risk of falls.

Wet bathroom floors are a leading cause of falls, so dry off the patient's feet before they leave the shower and provide a bath mat or rug with a rubber backing.

When walking outside, especially if the ground is wet, always hold the patient's arm.

Unfortunately, sleeping pills and anti-psychotic medications quadruple the risk of falling in the night. Be sure all hallways to the bathroom are well lit.

Floors must be clear of junk, shoes, pet toys, or other items that might cause the patient to trip or lose her balance. Alzheimer's patients who are hoarders—or are married to hoarders—have the greatest risk for falls. Get rid of piles of junk, even if the patient protests. (You can put her stuff in storage and tell her it is available should she ever need it. I have found most hoarders are more okay with their stuff being put in storage, they just can't handle having it thrown away or given to Goodwill.)

CHAPTER 25

EXPLOITATION AND MAINTAINING DIGNITY
Dr. Sally Burbank

Be aware! Shysters will crawl out of the woodwork ready to suck money out of trusting, cognitively-impaired senior adults. The cases I report below are those shared with me by the children of dementia patients.

Television Lures

Betty D. reported that her mother maxed out four credit cards buying junk from television infomercials before Betty found out and cancelled the cards. Betty, who lived a thousand miles away, had come to visit her mother after not seeing her for six months. When she arrived, she found the house filled with gadgets and items her eighty-nine-year-old mother neither needed nor had the space to store: a fancy food processor, a vegetable dehydrator, a smoothie Bullet, a set of cookware, an exercise contraption that was supposed to flatten the stomach, fancy necklaces and rings, dozens of jars of facial creams that worked "miraculously" to eliminate wrinkles. Most of the stuff was still in the box. Sadly, her mother had tried to assemble the pieces of the food processor but lacked the cognitive skills to follow the instructions.

All told, her mother had rung up over five thousand dollars on credit cards because she fell for every word the television salesperson said. When instructed to dial 1-800-BUY-THIS-GADGET, she'd dutifully obeyed, believing she couldn't live without the newest gizmo or wrinkle cream.

Moral of the story? Once patients have proven themselves unable to manage their finances, you should take away all credit and debit cards. AD patients can be very trusting and may be lured by the convincing spiels of attractive salesclerks.

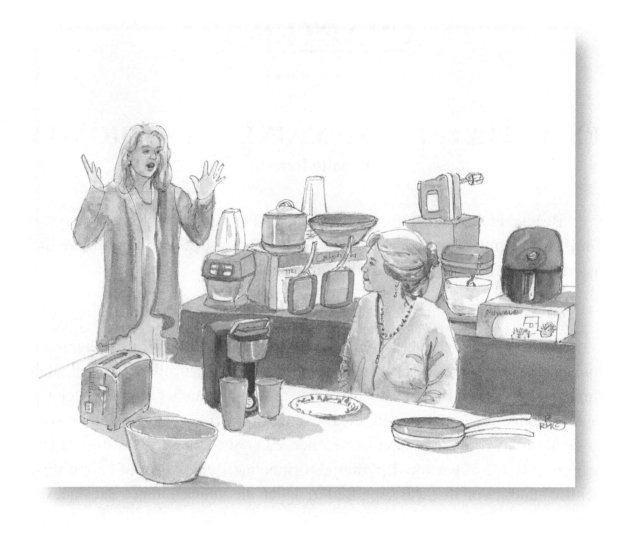

Con Artists

When Brad S. showed up at his elderly father's house to take him out for lunch, he noticed an unlabeled, white pick-up truck in the driveway. When he walked into the house, he discovered a "roofer" who had convinced his father the roof was in deplorable condition. The con man claimed the roof would cave in and the whole house would be damaged by the next big rainstorm if he didn't fix it immediately. Just as Brad walked in, his father had agreed to go to the bank and take out $5,000 in cash—the amount the "roofer" claimed he needed for the repair.

When Brad probed further and asked the "roofer" to show him the damaged shingles (and, while you're at it, a business card with a name and phone number, please!), the man presented several tattered shingles that were not even from his father's house!

The supposed roofer was caught red-handed and hurried away before the police could arrive. His truck conveniently had its license plate covered, so Brad could not take down the numbers. The police informed Brad this same man had swindled several other seniors into handing over money for a similar "must-do-now" roofing job. In every case, the con artist had taken the money and run. If Brad hadn't shown up when he did, the thief would have gotten away with stealing $5,000 from his father.

Online Scams

Online scammers routinely send emails professing they are from Bank of America or U.S. Bank or some other well-known institution. They claim the patient's account has been hacked and needs immediate attention. "Please update your billing information today by clicking this link…" The logos look identical to that of legitimate banks. I have nearly fallen for these scams myself but decided to bring my laptop to the bank and ask before divulging sensitive information. In every case, the email was from a scammer, not the bank. Seniors are especially prone to falling for such schemes. The scammer then gains entry into their bank accounts or steal their identity.

Family Members

Sadly, sometimes the thieves are not strangers, but family members. Margaret M. was beside herself when she discovered her nephew, a deadbeat drug abuser with no job, had regularly been visiting her mother and offering up sob stories about needing money for car repairs and gas to drive to work or he would lose his job. (The job he didn't have!) Turns out, the kid had conned Margaret's mother out of several thousand dollars over the course of a year. He would find the checkbook, write the check, and have his grandmother sign it. Since Margaret's mother survived only on a monthly Social Security check, she could ill-afford to support a drug-addicted grandson who was unmotivated to get a job or seek help for his drug problem. The rest of the family had long ago wised up and stopped enabling him. They couldn't believe he had stooped so low as to exploit his own grandmother when he knew she was poor and suffering from dementia.

Take home message? Talk personally to the bank officers where your loved one banks. If you have financial POA, they can put an alert on the account that allows the patient to take out no more than fifty dollars at a time and requires checks over $50 to be co-signed by you. If you live nearby, take away ATM cards and have bills paid through automatic withdrawals or with on-line banking that you control. Divvy out a set amount of money each week to cover the basics.

Many AD patients want control over their money, so bring them to the store with you each week and let them pay for their purchases. Let them have the satisfaction of plunking down the dollar bills and putting the change back in their wallet. Oversee the transaction carefully so your loved one isn't short-changed.

If the patient starts bouncing checks and living outside her means, give someone in the family who is trustworthy and responsible the financial power of attorney—a legal document that authorizes one person to act on behalf of another—in handling finances.

Exploitation by Caregiver

Unfortunately, some caregivers may not be trustworthy, as in this case:

Bev N. convinced her mother with moderate-stage AD to give her financial power of attorney. While most family members do an admirable job looking out for their parent's best interests, Bev squandered her mother's money by buying expensive furniture, a backyard pool, a trip to Florida, and even a pricey new Lexus. Bev claimed the pool allowed her mother to get some exercise, even though Mother showed little interest in swimming and didn't even own a swimsuit. Bev claimed she needed the new car to drive her mother to and from the doctor, even though her mother owned an old but reliable Camry. The Florida vacation was supposedly for Mom's benefit.

Meanwhile, Mom had no idea her sizable 401-k was being squandered by the very person she had entrusted to manage her money.

Douglas, a patient of mine, began investigating when he noticed his mother's bank account and 401-k balances had nose-dived without explanation. That's when he discovered his sister, Bev, had misappropriated the funds for things his mother didn't need.

When confronted, Bev became defensive. "I've done way more for Mom than you ever have, and I deserve a reward for all the hours I've spent driving Mom to the doctor and drug store and grocery store." Bev even went on to add, "Besides, I'll get half the money when Mom dies anyway, so why should I have to wait until she's dead to buy the stuff I need?"

Douglas was appalled. A luxury car and a swimming pool were a need? He took his sister to court to get the power of attorney revoked. Bev now refuses to have anything to do with her brother, but at least the mother's money won't run out before she dies.

Respect and Dignity

Prior to their diagnosis, AD patients had unique personalities and talents. Many raised loving families, excelled in their careers, became skilled cooks, golfers, or musicians. After the diagnosis, they progressively become forgetful and needy. But despite their growing dependence, they still deserve to be treated with respect, kindness, and dignity. Alzheimer's patients deserve the same care and affection we provide to babies and toddlers who are also dependent. Here are some ways you can show respect:

- Speak with a pleasant tone and use words that are understandable.
- Give only one direction or command at a time.
- Be cheerful and make the situation enjoyable whenever you can. Remember, the AD patient will mirror your mood.
- Find humor whenever you can.

- Never tell a patient how worn-out or burdened you feel taking care of them. They need to know they are loved and not a burden. Don't guilt trip them about all the extra work you must do because of their dependency. Trust me: they would far rather be living independently with a fully functioning brain, even if it meant doing their own laundry!

- Avoid arguing near or with the patient unless it is a matter of safety.

- Remind yourself when the AD patient acts out or does something totally out of character that they are operating with a diseased brain. It's the disease, not the patient. They are doing the best they can with what they have to work with. Try your hardest to be patient with them.

- Pick activities that don't require memory. For example, I used to look at seed catalogs with my father and ask him which tomatoes or flowers he liked best. As a retired farmer, he loved looking at gardening catalogs and would advise me on which species to purchase. Books showing colorful birds or flowers are things grandchildren can do with their grandparent. You don't have to remember the name of a bird or flower to appreciate its beauty.

- Find activities that the patient can do to help around the house. This will help her feel like she is contributing to the family. It could be washing a bathroom mirror, pairing socks, or deadheading the spent flowers in the flowerbox. Thank her for the help and tell her how much you appreciate her assistance. We all like to feel appreciated and needed.

- Remember to touch, pat, and hug your loved one often. Tell him you love him every day.

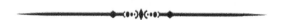

CHAPTER 26

•⟨••⟩◆⟨••⟩•

LEGAL MATTERS
Sue Bell and Dr. Sally Burbank

Wills

A will should delineate what is to become of a patient's material possessions at the time of death. A well-written will can prevent family squabbles. If a loved one has recently been diagnosed with AD, and they do not have a will, don't delay: get it done while the patient is still able to make rational decisions.

A will should consider the patient's many assets: houses, land, cars, personal belongings, financial accounts, and other worldly goods. Since the majority of AD patients are over sixty, many have accumulated a lifetime of possessions. Depending on how detailed you want to get, a will can divvy up even the smallest specialty items, such as jewelry, antiques, or family heirlooms.

While many elders espouse splitting everything up equally amongst the children, such an approach does not guarantee there will be no family quarrels. In my twenty-nine years of practice, I have known families to take each other to court, engage in fist fights, and even sneak into their mother's house to take valuables while the rest of the siblings were at the calling hours! I have seen siblings refuse to talk to each other because of disagreements over a parent's piano or riding lawn mower. In each case, the aggrieved sibling will tell me something like, "I can't believe my own sister would act like this. Mama was barely cold in the grave, and my sister went after the spoils."

One way to prevent these family feuds is to take photos of special items and attach the photos to a written list of what is to be given to specific family members. A person I know who was diagnosed with a terminal illness did this with her jewelry, making sure each child's share was equal. No matter how the will is drawn up, the end result should be that the items get to the right person. When it's set down in writing with pictures, there is less chance of argument.

A will should also spell out how to handle final arrangement expenses—coffin, tombstone, cemetery plot versus cremation—and it should name an executor.

Living Wills

A living will is a legal document that states a person's wishes concerning medical care once he or she is no longer able to make such decisions. The document should spell out the patient's desire for prolonging or not prolonging life through such means as feeding tubes, CPR, ventilators, and other life support systems. It can also specify whether or not to donate body organs.

Sample Directives from a Living Will

1. I direct my attending physician to withhold or withdraw life-sustaining medical care and treatment that is serving only to prolong the process of my dying if I should be in an incurable or irreversible mental or physical condition with no reasonable medical expectation of recovery.

2. I direct that treatment be limited to measures which are designed to keep me comfortable and to relieve pain, including any pain which might occur from the withholding or withdrawing of life-sustaining medical care or treatment.

In situations where there is no living will, family members are called upon to make the decisions. Often times, there are differing opinions, so conflicts often arise. Have this discussion about end of life decisions with the patient as early as possible.

The living will should be presented to doctors and hospitals and should be kept handy at all times. Forms for living wills are available from many senior service organizations, hospitals, doctors' offices, or they can be downloaded from the Internet.

In Tennessee, a living will becomes a legal document with the signature of the patient and two non-family witnesses. **A notary public or lawyer is NOT required.** This can vary from state to state. The patient's doctor will know the requirements for your state.

The patient needs to be of sound mind to complete a living will, so complete this document as soon as the diagnosis is made.

Power of Attorney

A power of attorney is a document that allows one individual (the agent) to act on behalf of another (the grantor). It can grant limited authority, such as making medical decisions or having control over a specific checking account, or it can grant broad authority over all the patient's financial and legal matters. The grantor is allowed to set boundaries and limits on what actions can be taken by the agent, such as stating which properties can be sold, how much the agent can spend on gift-giving, or how much the agent can be paid for services rendered.

A power of attorney should only be given to a trustworthy person who is willing and able to carry out the patient's wishes. This responsibility can be time-consuming, so select someone who has the time, intelligence and administrative skills.

When the patient is ready to sign over power of attorney, a simple legal document can be drafted in a lawyer's office, or forms can be downloaded from the internet, completed by the patient, and then signed by a notary public.

If the AD patient is incapable of handling his or her own affairs and yet refuses to grant power of attorney, the courts may have to intervene and declare the patient mentally incompetent. This requires statements from two doctors to be presented before a judge. If there is no family available to oversee the patient's welfare, a court-appointed guardian can be assigned. This person will charge a hefty fee for services, so it is best to choose a trusted family member, if possible.

Get a signed POA document when the patient is still in the early stages of Alzheimer's. All AD patients will eventually need someone to handle their affairs (unless they die of some other disease first). Even if the patient insists he is competent to handle his own affairs, he won't remain that way indefinitely.

To avoid the hassles of going to court or dealing with expensive lawyers or court-appointed guardians, don't delay getting this done. Emphasize to the patient that the POA won't take effect until the patient is mentally incompetent, and it is not a matter of *if* the patient becomes incapable of managing his affairs, it is a matter of *when*. If the patient won't listen to you, see if the patient's trusted doctor can convince him to get this done.

Driver's Licenses

Restricting the privilege of driving from someone with AD means a loss of independence for both the patient and the caregiver. This is one of the most emotional situations a caregiver will likely encounter. It's necessary, however, because, if the AD patient is involved in an accident for which he is liable, the patient's entire life savings and assets could be put in jeopardy. One man told me the hardest thing he did was take the car keys from his father, who broke down and wept. Though he knew he had to do it, it broke his heart to see his father sobbing.

What are the indications that a patient could put himself or others in danger if he continues to drive?

Signs that Driving Privileges Must Be Revoked:

- Running off the side of the road or hitting a mailbox or landing in the ditch.
- Weaving erratically, driving in the middle of the road or on the wrong side of the road.

- Running stop signs or forgetting that left turns must yield to oncoming traffic. Not yielding at yield signs or stopping at red lights.
- Driving so slowly other drivers honk or tailgate.
- Making poor decisions about what road and weather conditions are safe to drive in. Forgetting to wear a winter coat in freezing winter weather.
- Pulling out in front of cars. Not stopping for school busses or crosswalks.
- Getting lost driving home from familiar places.
- Difficulty backing out of the driveway or pulling into parking spaces.
- Repeatedly locking the keys in the car or leaving the car running.

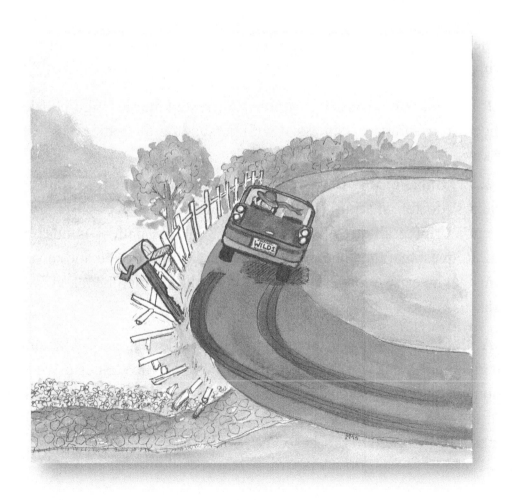

Most patients are already in the middle stage of AD before they are diagnosed, so this means that steps concerning driving may have to be taken immediately. Unfortunately, the issue of taking away the keys often isn't addressed until the patient has already had a fender bender or gotten lost. I recommend riding in the car on multiple occasions while your loved one is driving to get an honest assessment of their abilities. Some people give up the car keys easily. Women often have less trouble giving them up than men, especially when men are retired and have lots of time on their hands.

Research indicates that reasoning works most of the time, so a discussion should be the first step taken: it is often all that is needed. Begin by talking about the safety of the patient and others. If a close friend or family member has previously been in a car wreck, this makes understanding easier. Stress that you know they would never want to hurt anyone. If reasoning does not work, try the following:

1.   **Ask an authority figure.** A trusted public figure, such as a policeman or minister, can assist with persuading the patient to give up the car keys.

2.   **Engage the patient's trusted doctor.** Write a letter to the patient's doctor sharing specific behaviors you have observed of the patient's driving abilities that make you think the patient is unsafe on the road. Request that the doctor tell the patient in front of you and in very clear terms that he can no longer drive. The keys should then be taken away. End of discussion!

A professional truck driver was in the middle stages of Alzheimer's when he was diagnosed, and the doctor told him he could no longer drive. The driver went home and threw his keys in a desk drawer. His wife said he would go out, sit in the truck, and take naps for two or three hours, but he never tried to drive again. Doctor's orders worked in this case.

3. **Ask your insurance agent.** A detailed explanation of the hazards and liabilities associated with driving when it is no longer safe may get through to the patient.

4. **Get the patient's driving abilities formally tested.** This can be done at the state government's licensing facility (Dept. of Safety or Dept. of Motor Vehicles) or at a driving school. An objective driving test performed by someone other than yourself can prove the patient is no longer a safe driver without you being the "bad guy."

5. **Give the car to a child or grandchild.** Tell the AD patient that the family member desperately needs the car to get to work or college but will return it "soon."

6. **If all else fails, disable the car.** Remove the battery or take the keys and lock them up! One wife took some liberties with the truth when she told her husband the car "needed work" and could not be driven until the mechanic ordered the appropriate part. Since Alzheimer's patients have a poor ability to judge how much time has elapsed, he didn't notice the mechanic had already taken six months to get the part!

7. **Lock up the car keys.** (And spare keys!) If you, the caregiver, are still driving, you may need to take extraordinary measures to keep the keys secured. Let him vent and yell, then calmly inform him, "I know it is upsetting to not be able to drive anymore, but I want you safe and alive." Stay calm and don't argue—but don't cave in! Don't let him guilt-trip you into letting him drive.

Whatever method you use, don't forget that the patient won't remember these controversies. *You* are the one who will feel guilty, but you would feel much worse if the patient got into an accident and killed someone. If there is a blessing with this disease, it is that the patient's short-term memory makes any disagreements quickly forgotten.

~ Safety takes precedence over a patient's desire to drive! ~

―――

Car Rides and Living in the Moment

My husband, Ray, was particularly strong-minded, but we found that his desire to drive was satisfied by going on long rides together. We would journey each afternoon throughout the countryside in our town, which he really enjoyed. Many AD patients don't particularly want to run errands, but they do want to ride around—sometimes for hours on end. If someone volunteers to help, ask them to take the patient on a joy ride. Be sure to reimburse the cost of the volunteer's gas and remind them to lock the car doors so the patient won't try to get out of the moving vehicle.

In the beginning, as we rode for a couple of hours each afternoon, Ray would get excited and point to sights along the way. "Look at the horse," or, "That's a big tree," or "Those are pretty flowers." As the disease progressed, he would just point to items wanting me to see and acknowledge them. In the end, he just sat quietly and enjoyed the ride. He never quit wanting to go on rides the entire nine years he had AD.

Long rides on back roads are especially suited for patients with AD because they can live in the moment and enjoy the sights. They don't need a good memory to enjoy pretty flowers, unusual houses, or horses.

Remember this basic rule in any difficult situation: Always treat the patient with kindness and respect. The old adage that honey gathers more flies than vinegar is true. Gentle words work well because AD patients are in a world of feeling and emotion. This goes a long way in convincing the patient to give up the car keys. Remind them you want them to give up the car keys because you love and care about them, not to punish them.

Transportation Options

When the patient can no longer drive, someone else will have to chauffeur them, which can be a time-consuming burden for the caregiver. It is therefore helpful to identify others who can assist with driving if you are at work or unavailable.

Most caregivers enlist friends, family, church members, and neighbors to assist. Be sure to cover the volunteer's gas and time. Don't exploit these angels by expecting them to pay for the gas to transport your mother to the doctor. Pay them generously if you want them to help you again!

One caregiver found a taxi driver she knew on a first-name basis and fully trusted. She kept his phone number handy and trusted him to take her mother to appointments and to escort her inside. The taxi driver arranged for the hair stylist or doctor to call him once Mother was ready to be picked up. The taxi driver appreciated having a reliable client, and the caregiver appreciated the extra attention he provided to safely escort Mother to her appointments and get her safely in the house. The caregiver provided a generous tip to cover the extra time and attention he provided. Perhaps a similar arrangement could be made with a local Uber or Lyft driver or a retired neighbor wanting a little extra spending money.

If you cannot locate someone you know to bring Mom to the doctor, call **Eldercare at 1 (800) 677-1116,** and they can assist with finding a volunteer or paid driver in your area. You can also call the National Aging Network in your county, or the Alzheimer's Association in your state for further assistance.

In June of 2018, Congress passed **CHRONIC** (Creating High-quality Results and Outcomes Necessary to Improve Chronic Care). This bill will allow Medicare Advantage plans (but NOT plain Medicare) to provide transportation to doctor's appointments. When the Medicare enrollment period comes in November of each year, perhaps you could select an Advantage plan that offers this benefit. Advantage plans include BC/BS Advantage, Humana, and Healthspring. Do your homework, as the plan is not *required* to provide transportation, but Medicare will cover it if they do. Ask to speak with the "Care Coordinator" if your loved one is on an Advantage plan and request that the patient be provided transportation to the doctor through the CHRONIC bill passed by Congress in June of 2018. Perhaps if enough patients demand the service, the Advantage plan will provide the drivers.

CHAPTER 27

━●━‹•··›‹•··›━●━

Working with Doctors

Dr. Sally Burbank

One of the challenging aspects of caregiving a loved one with Alzheimer's disease is deciding how aggressive to be with the patient's other medical issues. For example, let's say your husband with moderate Alzheimer's disease is told he needs a pacemaker because his heartrate drops dangerously low or that he needs a cardiac bypass surgery due to heart blockages. Or what if an orthopedic doctor recommends the patient have a knee replacement because his knee has bone-on-bone arthritis, or the gastroenterologist informs you it is time for a ten-year colonoscopy screening?

What do you do? How aggressive should you be? You don't want to appear uncaring, or worse—like you're too anxious to collect his life insurance money! Will the specialist label you "non-compliant" or "difficult" if you do not go along with every recommendation?

Your gut tells you not to put your loved one through major surgery, but then self-doubt kicks in. Who are you to question a doctor? Secretly, however, you are telling yourself, "If we put in a pacemaker or cardiac stent, aren't we just keeping him alive that much longer? And for what? So that his memory can go from bad to worse until he finally winds up clueless and barely able to swallow in five years? Why would I do anything to prolong his life when Alzheimer's is a disease with a guaranteed downward trajectory?"

These are difficult questions, so let's think it through.

Specialists are geared to focus on their area of expertise, not the well-being of the person as a whole. The gastroenterologist may not grasp the severity of your loved one's dementia, largely because you ensure the patient shows up for the doctor's appointment freshly bathed, fed, and properly attired. In addition, many patients are able to hide their cognitive deficiencies surprisingly well during a brief office visit, especially if the spouse or daughter takes over answering the questions. Also, many caregivers are reluctant to embarrass their loved one by "ratting" on them to the doctor or nurse about the patient's cognitive problems right in front of the patient.

What should you do?

I recommend handing the nurse a short note describing the severity of dementia and asking her to read it and share it with the doctor. This will alert the doctor before the office visit, and he or she may be less likely to suggest aggressive surgeries or treatments. Also, if forewarned, the doctor will know to look more carefully for signs of Alzheimer's disease.

If you want the doctor to see how bad the AD really is, after you've handed over the note, allow the *patient* the opportunity to answer the doctor's questions. Too often the spouse or daughter butts in and answers the questions rather than making the patient stumble for words, and thereby reveal the severity of the illness. Let the doctor see for themselves that your mother or husband can't answer any of the questions. Be forewarned! AD patients will sometimes make up answers or say what they think the doctor wants to hear rather than admit they cannot remember. In the note, ask the doctor to ask open-ended questions where the patient has to answer with a sentence, and not just a "yes" or "no." Questions such as, "What did you eat for breakfast?" (not, "Did you eat a healthy breakfast?") will better reveal the cognitive decline.

Family practitioners and internists are trained to provide a total body assessment and a long-term view, so if you are unsure whether to perform a particular surgery or procedure recommended by a specialist, bring your loved one in for a second opinion to the primary care doctor who knows the patient best. Schedule an actual appointment rather than trying to get your questions handled by telephone or email, as the doctor needs to see for him/herself how bad the patient is. The question to ask the doctor is, "What are the pros and cons of doing what Dr. So-and-So recommends?" The next question is equally important: "Dr. Smith, if this were *your* mother with this stage of AD, would you do it?"

Remember, just because a specialist says your loved one qualifies for a knee replacement, pacemaker, or prostate cancer surgery, it doesn't mean you have to do it! In fact, aggressive treatment often turns out to be a huge mistake with AD patients. Why?

Time spent in the hospital is bewildering and frightening to Alzheimer's patients. They often can't remember why they are there, who all the unfamiliar nurses and doctors are, or why people want to repeatedly jab needles in their arm and wake them up to check their blood pressure. They may sundown, get belligerent, and holler at night. They frequently yank out their IVs and urine catheters. They often refuse to swallow the pills the nurses provide and will instead squirrel them in their cheeks and spit them out when the nurse turns her back. In the worst cases, I have seen agitated AD patients assault an unsuspecting nurse or physical therapist if the patient thinks the staff member is badgering them.

Some will wander the halls completely lost. They will forget their room number and enter the wrong room, startling other patients. Some forget why they got out of bed in the first place. When the nursing staff asks what they need, they don't remember. More disturbing, AD patients can climb over bedrails and fall.

While the nursing staff does its best to keep track of all patients, Alzheimer's patients have an uncanny ability to escape in the thirty seconds a nurse is distracted by another patient. Be sure the nurses know your loved one has AD. Request a room closest to the nursing station, if possible, so the staff can keep a better eye on your loved one. Patients at the end of the hall nearest the elevator are the most likely to wander off.

If you ever have to leave your demented family member alone at night, speak personally with the charge nurse and notify her when you are leaving so she will know to check in on your loved one more frequently. If you are too exhausted to stay the night and can't find anyone else, hire someone to stay. Hospitals are understaffed, and there simply aren't enough nurses to provide one-on-one care for your loved one (unless they are in the intensive care unit). The average night nurse may have twelve patients for whom she has to administer medications, document vitals, and observe for medical problems. Add to that the cumbersome but mandatory electronic documentation, and you can see why the average nurse cannot sit in your loved one's room keeping him out of trouble—if she spends a lot of time with your loved one, she is neglecting the others.

Restraints

In days gone by, family members would frequently walk into their loved one's hospital room in the morning only to discover Dad tied to the bed with a Posey vest or wrist restraints to keep him from falling out of bed, pulling out his IVs, or wandering off. The patient's arms would often be covered with bruises from repeated attempts to escape the restraints. Families would be furious to see their father tied up like an animal. Patients found these experiences terrifying.

Without restraints, however, demented patients frequently crawled over the bedrails and broke a hip. They pulled out their IVs, nasogastric tubes, or urine catheters, causing trauma and bleeding. Greedy lawyers then lined up to sue hospitals for allowing this "neglect" to happen.

Demented patients often get disoriented, agitated, argumentative, and combative, and their incessant hollering disturbs other patients who are trying to sleep. When in this state, they cannot be reasoned with. Some pull their surgical bandages off and pick at their stitches, causing bleeding and infection.

By morning, however, the patient will often transform back into a model patient. When the nurse tries to tell the family what a rough night she had, the patient will lie in bed angelically, seemingly the perfect patient. Dr. Jekyll and Mr. Hyde! After a few hours, however, the patient becomes sleepy from his restless night and wants to sleep all day. Attempts to keep him awake to eat or take his medications only makes him crotchety and uncooperative.

Your loved one won't remember the important things the nurse tries to tell him. She may scold him repeatedly for picking at his surgical dressing, but the message is forgotten within five minutes. If the nurse puts on Posey mitts to keep him from picking, he may fall trying to get out of bed. In short, hospital stays for

---

patients with Alzheimer's are a lose-lose proposition for everyone—except perhaps the sue-hungry attorneys who advertise on city buses!

The Take-Home Message? A family member should stay in the hospital room day and night to ensure an Alzheimer's patient's safety. Expect a rotten night of sleep unless sedating medications are given to the patient. It can help to sit next to the patient's bed and hold her hand. Talk soothingly until she falls asleep. One daughter sang her mother's favorite hymns to calm her at night. Hire a private sitter if you need time away, but never leave her alone in the room at night, or bad things can happen.

Anesthesia

Anesthesia and potent narcotic pain medications tax the already limited brain capacity of AD patients. They trigger agitation and confusion, and, not infrequently, hallucinations. Even worse, most caregivers report that after general anesthesia, the patient's cognitive function—already limited—takes a nosedive and may never return to its pre-hospitalization level. In short, every time an AD patient gets general anesthesia, the brain takes a "hit" from which the patient may never fully recover.

Elective Surgeries

For all the reasons stated above, surgery, anesthesia, pain medications, and hospitalizations are extremely traumatic for Alzheimer's patients and families. Worse, the patient often suffers a major drop in cognitive function. My advice? Say no to elective surgeries whenever possible.

Feeding Tubes

As AD progresses and the patient no longer eats enough to maintain a healthy weight, well-meaning doctors, nurses, and family members may push to insert a feeding tube. "You don't want her to starve to death, do you?" I've heard people say.

Feeding tubes are ALWAYS a bad idea in late-stage Alzheimer's. Many times, the demented individual will pull out or fiddle with the tube, causing trauma, stomach perforation, or infection. Worse, the liquid nutrition (tube feed) often gets aspirated into the patient's lungs causing pneumonia.

While feeding tubes make caregivers fret less about a loved one's weight, it does nothing for the well-being of the patient. The Alzheimer's patient is on a downward trajectory to die. Does it really matter whether she weighs ninety pounds or one hundred twenty pounds when she does?

Assuage your guilt with the following proven fact: Alzheimer's patients don't experience hunger in the way we do. When they are hungry, they eat—if offered easy-to-chew-and-swallow foods that they like. Your job is to provide healthy, easy-to-eat meals and frequent snacks they need. Let Mom eat as much as she wants, whenever she wants.

In late-stage AD, however, you will have to spoon-feed your patient at every meal, as she won't remember how to eat. Often, the rapid weight loss seen in nursing homes is because a dinner tray is left at the patient's bedside, but nobody takes the twenty minutes at every meal to spoon-feed the patient. AD patients eat very slowly, and frankly, nursing homes don't have enough staff members to hand feed each one. Plus, in late-stage AD, the patient is asleep up to twenty hours a day. Hence, they lose weight.

Not a single study shows feeding tubes prolong life or improve cognitive function or quality of life. In fact, they just seem to agitate the patient. I do not recommend inserting a feeding tube in an attempt to prolong a loved one's life: you may just *shorten* it by inducing aspiration pneumonia or a hole in the patient's stomach.

Medications

What about the long list of medications so many Alzheimer's patients wind up on? Are they necessary?

Most elderly patients see four to five specialists, and it seems each one wants to prescribe a couple medications. My advice is to stay off any drug that aggravates cognitive function—pain meds, sleeping pills, Benadryl, muscle relaxers, incontinence meds. Be sure to keep blood pressure in excellent control because mini-strokes—or worse yet, massive strokes caused by poorly controlled hypertension—will worsen cognitive function. Even meds designed to *treat* Alzheimer's can have side effects of dizziness, sedation, confusion, and nausea.

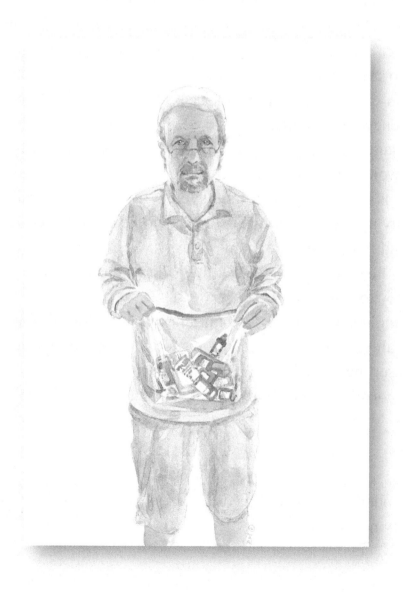

Caregivers should sit down with the patient's internist or family practitioner to review every drug, herb, and vitamin with the question, "Is this drug absolutely necessary for a patient with dementia?" Another important questions? "Could this drug aggravate Mom's dementia, poor appetite, or agitation?" This is a critical discussion because the cognitive side effects of many medications are even more pronounced in those who are already cognitively impaired.

I tell all my elderly patients to bring a bag with the bottle of every drug, supplement, and herb the patient takes (not just a list with the names of the drugs) to their office visits. I then personally review each bottle and write out a schedule of exactly which drugs to take at breakfast, lunch, supper, and bedtime. Some of my patients get these medication schedules laminated. To encourage compliance, I try to minimize how many times a day a patient must take medications. Purchase a pill dispenser (sometimes called a medication caddy or pill organizer) clearly labeled with the days of the week, and fill it weekly, based on the schedule written out by the doctor.

In summary, decisions about the risks and benefits of any given surgery, treatment, or medication should be thoughtfully reviewed and discussed with the patient's primary care doctor. Try to avoid overnight hospital stays, and instead of general anesthesia, ask if local anesthetic blocks (axillary, spinal, epidural) could be used instead. Seek a second opinion on all non-emergency surgeries with the patient's primary care doctor, as he or she knows your loved one best.

Effect of Medications on Cognitive Function

The cognitive side effects of medications are exacerbated in patients with Alzheimer's disease, as they don't have the brain reserve to withstand even the slightest "hit" to the brain. Pain pills, sleeping pills, Parkinson's meds, Benadryl, urinary incontinence medications like oxybutynin—all cross into the brain and aggravate confusion, agitation, and sedation.

Even drugs designed to treat AD can cause problems. I once tried an Alzheimer's patient on the lowest dose of Aricept, a drug that is supposed to help delay the decline in memory. Her caregiver called me the next week, stating her mother was dizzy and sleeping day and night. In her case, we had to stop it. Thus, the first thing I do with many Alzheimer's patients is STOP any drug that is not essential.

Medication Doses

Many new patients come in with a grocery bag full of herbs, vitamins, and medications, each prescribed by a small army of specialists. Each specialist is looking at the one body part they specialize in (clogged heart, leaky bladder, bum knee, tremor, drippy nose), but no one is looking at the brain! No one seems to consider the *cumulative* effects of mixing all these herbs and medications.

More and more, we physicians are learning about drug interactions and the cumulative result of combining all these pills. Many times, the caregiver correctly surmises that her ninety-pound, eighty-five-year-old mother is overmedicated. Unfortunately, most caregivers don't question the doctor: they just assume the doctor knows best.

The patient's primary care doctor is most equipped to evaluate the patient as a whole and eliminate all drugs that are not 100 percent essential. The most common medications that aggravate cognitive function include:

- Pain pills (hydrocodone, oxycodone, tramadol, oxycontin)
- Sleeping pills (amitriptyline, zolpidem, temazepam, trazodone)
- Muscle relaxers (cyclobenzaprine)
- Anti-depressants (citalopram, escitalopram, Paxil, Remeron, trazodone)
- Incontinence drugs (oxybutynin, Ditropan)
- Allergy medications (Benadryl, Zyrtec, Hydroxyzine)
- Anxiety medications (alprazolam, clonazepam, lorazepam, diazepam)
- Parkinson's medications (Sinemet, carbidopa/levodopa)
- Alzheimer's disease medications (Aricept, Exelon, Namzaric)

Unfortunately, all too often, these are the very drugs patients or family members insist the patient cannot live without! "She won't sleep a wink without her Ambien, Dr. Burbank," I am frequently told. Or, "She has to have her pain pills, or she'll moan all night." Families seem fine with stopping the cholesterol, blood pressure, and diabetes pills, but "Don't you dare touch her nerve pill!"

Unfortunately, these "can't-live-without-them" drugs are the very ones that aggravate patients' cognition. Thus, I try to wean them off these drugs, which is not an easy task, especially if they have been taking sleep, nerve, or pain pills for decades! I am always unpopular when I push to stop these medications.

Medications for Treating Alzheimer's

Doctors sometimes recommend medications to treat AD. Although no drug can cure or reverse memory loss, there are medications that slow the progression of the disease. In fact, currently available drugs can delay late-stage disease or the need for a nursing home by about six months. While this may not seem like much, the longer a patient stays in mild to moderate AD, the longer they will be able to independently handle activities of daily living, such as bathing, toileting, dressing and eating. This frees up the caregiver's time and may allow patients to live in their own homes longer.

The most common AD drug, Aricept, is now available in the generic form donepezil. This drug is often prescribed in combination with Namenda (generic name memantine). There is now a drug that combines these two medications called Namzaric. This combo drug is more effective than either drug by itself, but it is not available in generic form and costs over $400 per month. For this reason, I usually prescribe donepezil and memantine as two separate drugs, unless the patient's Part D drug coverage makes Namzaric affordable.

Alternative medications to donepezil include the Exelon patch (rivastigmine) or Razadyne (galantamine). The most common side effects include diarrhea, insomnia, decreased appetite, headache, sedation, dizziness, nausea, vomiting, and heart rhythm issues. Memantine can cause constipation, dizziness, and headache.

Discuss the risks versus benefits of Alzheimer medications with your doctor.

Pills for Sleep and Pain

Sleeping pills (like Ambien/zolpidem) and pain pills (like hydrocodone and oxycodone) quickly become habit forming, and soon, patients cannot fall asleep without the medication. This would not be a huge deal if studies didn't show that elderly patients on sleeping or pain pills have a quadrupled risk of falls and hip fractures compared to those NOT on them. The falls often happen at night when the patient gets up to go to the bathroom while under the influence of these sedating medications. Pain and sleep meds also worsen a patient's balance and reflexes. In a poorly lit bedroom, bathroom, or hallway, patients easily lose their balance and fall, or they trip over something and wind up on the floor with a fractured hip.

The consequences of sleeping pills and narcotic pain pills—especially when used together in elderly patients—have become so problematic that Medicare is no longer willing to pay for them. My patients bitterly complain about this, but Medicare's stance is, "Why should we pay for a drug proven to increase the risk of hip fractures, and then turn around and pay the high price of hip surgery, physical therapy, and rehab?"

It is often a battle to get elderly patients who have been taking sleeping pills or pain pills for decades to get off their medication. The real key to solving insomnia is to keep the patient from nodding off in their chair throughout the day. If they catnap even a few minutes, it may interfere with their sleep at night. Naps are fine, so long as the patient sleeps at night.

Keeping the patient awake and stimulated throughout the day, however, is a time and energy drain on the caregiver. Thus, it is often the caregiver that asks me to prescribe a pill to "knock Mother out so I can get some sleep." Melatonin and trazodone are frequently used and are safer than zolpidem or tranquillizers, but trazodone can have a hangover effect.

Coming to agreement about sleeping pills and pain pills in elderly patients is often the area where patients, caregivers, and doctors butt heads. Medicare slaps doctors on the wrist if we prescribe sleeping pills because of the increased hip fracture rates. Pain pills also increase the risk for hospitalization due to accidental overuse.

On the other hand, caregivers have trouble getting enough sleep if their demented parent or spouse roams the house making noise at night. If drugs seem absolutely necessary, use the lowest dose possible. Ten milligrams of zolpidem (Ambien) in an elderly woman is now deemed dangerously high: 2.5 or 5 mg is considered a more appropriate dose.

In the end, patients often get far fewer narcotic pain pills and sleeping pills than they would like, and we physicians cave in and prescribe more pills than we want to. If patients suffer significant pain and insomnia despite Tylenol and proper sleep hygiene (consistent bedtime, no caffeine after noon, no bright TV or computer screen for at least two hours before bed, no catnapping), we often acquiesce. Meaningful discussions with your primary care doctor are the only way to come to a consensus on balancing risks and benefits.

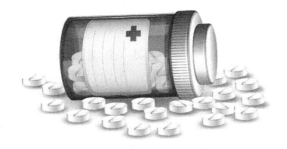

CHAPTER 28

PATIENT SAFETY
Sue Bell

How to Physically Handle a Patient

People with Alzheimer's disease sometimes need caregivers to physically assist them, especially as the disease progresses. Since the patient has difficulty communicating his needs, it can be difficult to determine how much assistance is required. Sometimes the patient may need help transitioning from one place to another, such as from the bed to a chair, getting in and out of a tub or automobile, or going up and down the stairs. They may also need help crossing the street safely.

When Assisting a Patient up from a Chair or Bed:

- Be aware their skin can be fragile.

- Don't pull on their arms or legs to get them up, as the joints can dislocate easily. Instead, lift under both armpits, or scoop them up under one armpit and around their back to the other armpit.

- You may need to use a draw sheet when turning them over in bed. A transfer board can help move them from a bed to a wheelchair. This is more comfortable for the patient and helps you avoid heavy lifting. Hospital beds also help you get the patient out of bed without straining your back.

- Arrange for a physical therapist to teach you how to lift and transfer a patient from the bed or chair without straining your back. Most patients are able to walk until the end stage, but some become frail and lose the ability to get out of the chair or bed, especially if they live into their nineties. I did not have to lift Ray at all the entire nine years he was alive as he could walk until the day he died.

- Hold onto the patient's hand or waistband while walking, especially if he is about to cross the street. This prevents him from stepping in front of a car. It also prevents him from going in the wrong direction.

- If the patient pulls his hand away, wrap your arm around his waist and hold onto the arm furthest away from you. Have him wrap his arm around your shoulder or waist.

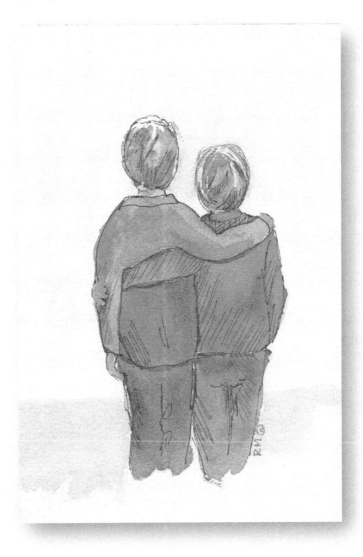

Equipment You May Find Useful:

Draw sheets, hospital beds, wheelchairs, walkers, bathing chairs that roll into showers, bedside potty chairs, potty chair liners, grab bars, portable raised toilet seats, a portable ramp for wheelchairs, hand rails for commodes and showers, a lift chair, chair aids that help the patient go from sitting to standing, and a transfer board. Physical and occupational therapists can help you sort out which aids will be most beneficial. Occupational therapists can assist with finding tools to make hygiene and eating easier. You can ask your primary care doctor to arrange a PT/OT consult. With a physician's order, Medicare will usually pay for needed medical equipment.

a. Walker with Seat

b. Grab Bar

c. Shower Chair

d. Wheelchair

e. Footed Cane

f. Portable Ramp

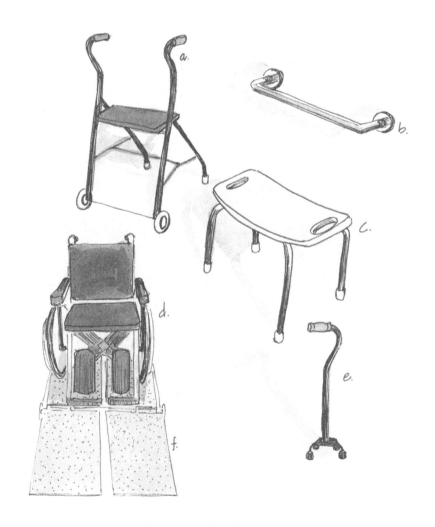

Safety at Home

As their AD advances, your loved one will eventually not understand the difference between safe and unsafe actions, so you will need to make changes in the home to reduce the chance of accidents. Examine the house room by room to assess potential dangers. Too often I've seen patients fall down stairs that have no railing. The response of the caregiver is, "I meant to have a railing installed."

~ Good intentions don't prevent accidents—action does! No excuses… Get it done! ~

Here are some simple safety measures to consider:

- Place childproof locks on cabinets where toxic chemicals and cleaners are stored. Bright-colored liquids such as detergents or Windex appeal to AD patients and can be harmful if swallowed or sprayed in the eyes.
- Make sure rooms that pose dangers have locks and alarms on them. Hang bells on doorknobs.
- Install dead bolts on the front and back doors that require a key and don't let the patient know where the key is kept. Combination locks may also be used. Write down the combinations so you don't forget them!
- Install battery-powered alarms on your outside doors—or, if you prefer, a full house alarm system—so the patient cannot leave without you being alerted. Make sure you keep the alarm system activated.
- Put safety caps (Grip and Twist Door Knob Covers) on doors leading to the outside or to off-limit rooms.
- Lock up sharp knives and small appliances such as blenders, mixers, and food processors in childproof cabinets.
- Keep chainsaws, electric trimmers, hedge clippers, and other power tools in a locked shed or room where the patient doesn't have a key. AD

patients are notorious for wanting to use the hedge trimmers or the lawn mower long past the time it is safe.

- Have cell phones and portable phones charged and handy at all times. Install locator apps on the phone.
- If the patient sleeps in a separate bedroom, install a baby monitor so the sounds you hear will alert you if they fall or if there is an emergency.
- Lock yourself and the patient in the house day and night to prevent your loved one from wandering off when you are in the bathroom.
- Put up baby gates to keep the patient from falling down stairs.
- Take the knobs off the stove when it isn't being used so the patient cannot turn the burners on when you are asleep.
- Install motion sensor night lights to illuminate the pathway when motion is detected. Many patients roam at night, and when it is dark, your loved one is more apt to bump into things, trip, and fall. You can also install dimmer switches on the lights, so you can leave lights at a low level. At the very least, insert nightlights.
- Hide the pet's food and water in an inconspicuous place like the laundry room. Patients have been known to eat Fido's food and water.
- Take all guns out of the house! AD patients forget safety procedures, and many a wife has walked in and found her husband fiddling with a loaded gun. Even if you hide or lock them up, AD patients have an uncanny ability to find them!
- Remove sharp knives and sharp-tipped scissors, especially if the patient has a tendency for temper tantrums and violence.
- Make sure all small, colorful, shiny objects like coins and marbles are removed. Patients may think they are candy and try to eat them.
- Don't give your loved one hard candy, suckers, or Jell-O, which are choking hazards. Sugar-free chewing gum is okay, and most patients will chew the gum for hours.

- When your patient puts something inappropriate in his mouth, do not try to take the item out with your finger. Like a dog with a desired bone, he will not give up the item in his mouth without a fight. Instead, insert a wooden spoon, turn it sideways and then remove the object.

- Remove all throw rugs from the floor, as they can cause the patient to slip or trip. Throw rugs are a leading cause of hip fractures.

- Put no-slip adhesives or a no-skid mat in the tub to prevent slipping. Install handrails or handholds at an appropriate height to get in and out of the tub.

- If the patient tends to fiddle with the thermostat and moves the temperature setting to unhealthy levels (one lady kept moving the thermostat to 90 degrees!), install a fake thermostat and have the real thermostat put in a hidden place. The patient can then "adjust" the temperature at will—without changing a thing.

Choking

As Alzheimer's disease progresses, the brain has difficulty communicating with the body on even the most basic bodily functions. Thus, in addition to losing bladder control, most patients in the last stage of the disease have difficulty swallowing, and they frequently choke. The medical term for this is dysphagia.

Signs of dysphagia include: reluctance or fear of eating, squirreling food in the cheeks instead of swallowing, coughing frequently when eating, choking spells, unexplained weight loss, and eating too fast.

Other medical conditions can cause dysphagia, so don't assume it is the AD. The dentist can examine the patient's mouth and gums for ulcers or dental problems. A gastroenterologist can determine if the esophagus has a stricture that causes food to get stuck. Strictures can be dilated in a simple, outpatient procedure. Also, your pharmacist can examine all medications to see if any of them cause a dry mouth, which makes swallowing difficult. Bottom line: You must be your patient's detective and try to figure out what is causing the difficulty.

Besides being frightening to both the patient and caregiver, choking can lead to aspiration of food into the lungs, which causes pneumonia. Even worse, AD patients can choke to death on a chunk of food lodged in their trachea.

If the dysphagia is due to AD, the caregiver must be extremely attentive when the patient eats. Mealtimes should be calm and quiet with a minimum of distractions. The patient should sit upright, preferably at a table. The food should be served at an appropriate temperature—not too hot or cold—and the food should be cut into small pieces. Stringy meats, like roast beef, are especially hazardous, so consider grinding them up and adding gravy. The mayonnaise in tuna or egg salad provides moisture and helps the food slide down. Thin, soft foods, such as applesauce, yogurt, cottage cheese, mashed potatoes, oatmeal, ice cream, canned peaches, and watermelon are easy to eat. Finger foods and eating with a spoon makes mealtime easier. Occupational therapists can assist with locating easy-to-grasp big-handled utensils. Some recommend a big-handled "spork."

Some patients squirrel away food in their cheeks. They keep eating and chewing but forget to swallow. You may have to remind the patient to swallow before taking another bite. Encouraging them to drink between bites can help. Eventually, your patient may have to be spoon-fed. This can be very time consuming, because AD patients often eat very slowly. Allow adequate time for meals so your patient isn't rushed and thereby tempted to swallow before the food is thoroughly chewed.

Patients sometimes have difficulty swallowing thin liquids like water or even their own saliva. Most pharmacies have, or can order, a product called Thicken. You stir this powder into water causing it to thicken slightly, making it easier to swallow. Milk and Ensure are easier to swallow than water. Perhaps when a liquid is thicker and has flavor, the mouth remembers to swallow. A small juice glass with only 2-3 ounces of liquid works best; it doesn't allow the patient to swallow too much at a time. Straws are also a good option, as they keep the patient from gulping, and they force the patient to swallow.

Eating became problematic for my mother when she reached end-stage Alzheimer's. She would forget how to swallow, and then she would choke. She aspirated food into her lungs many times. Choking terrified her, and a couple of times she choked so badly she turned blue.

My siblings and I met with the doctor to discuss whether a feeding tube should be placed. The doctor explained that most families feel guilty if they don't place a feeding tube because they think withholding nutrition is somehow "starving" their loved one. Studies show, however, that after three days without food or water, patients no longer feel hungry or thirsty, and they then go on to die peacefully of kidney failure over the course of several weeks. Mom's doctor did not recommend a feeding tube due to the risk of aspiration pneumonia and prolonging the inevitable. She had already become mute, bed-bound, and was now unable to swallow. She already slept up to twenty hours a day. Why would we want to prolong her life? To what end?

We listened to the doctor's advice, and after about ten days, she gradually fell into a coma and died peacefully, with no more terrifying spells of turning blue. Our family has never regretted our decision to withhold the feeding tube and let nature take its course.

Good Foods for Late-stage AD

Carnation Breakfast	Milkshakes
Ensure Plus or Boost Plus	Applesauce
Soft, cooked vegetables	Oatmeal
Scrambled eggs	Pureed meats
Mashed potatoes	Puddings
Creamy soups - no chunks	Cottage cheese
Macaroni and cheese	Yogurt

Jars of baby food provide a quick and easy food choice because they are naturally juicy and help prevent dehydration.

Taking Medications

In early AD, patients can usually still swallow their pills, but in the middle and later stages, pills and capsules become a choking hazard.

If the patient starts having trouble swallowing a medication, ask the patient's doctor if the medicine can be provided in a form that is easier to take, such as a liquid or capsule that can be opened and sprinkled, or perhaps in a gummy chew. If not, get a mortar and pestle and crush the tablets and stir them into a favorite food. Be sure and check with your doctor or pharmacist to make sure the medicine can be safely crushed or mixed with food. Various types of mortar and pestles are available online from Amazon.

Patients will spit out any medication that has a bitter taste. One way to mask the taste is to combine it with foods such as applesauce, mashed banana, or ice cream.

The Heimlich Maneuver ®

Learn the Heimlich maneuver so you won't feel powerless if your patient chokes. Remember, however, that this procedure should NOT be attempted as long as the patient is still coughing or able to speak. It should be reserved for when food is lodged so fully in the patient's trachea that he or she is unable to breathe (and may even be turning blue). The choking victim may put a hand to the throat, the universal sign that means, "I am choking!" Quick action is needed. A victim has only five minutes of not being able to breathe before brain damage starts.

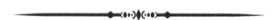

Heimlich Maneuver for a Standing Victim

1. From behind, wrap your arms around the choking victim's waist.

2. Make a fist and place the thumb side of your fist against the victim's upper abdomen, below the ribcage and just above the navel.

3. Grasp your fist with your other hand and press into the victim's abdomen with quick, upward pressure. Do not squeeze the ribcage; confine the force to the upward thrust of your hands. Repeat till the object is expelled.

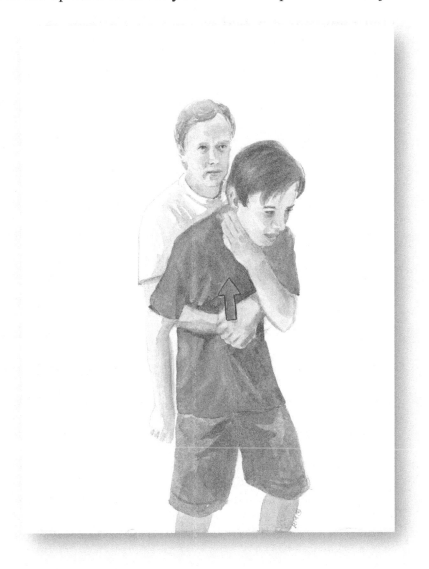

Heimlich Maneuver for an Unconscious Victim

1. Place victim on his back.

2. Kneel astride the victim's hips facing the victim.

3. With one hand on top of the other, place the heel of your bottom hand on the abdomen, below the rib cage and just above the navel.

4. Use your body weight to press into the victim's abdomen with a quick, upward pressure.

5. Repeat until object is expelled.

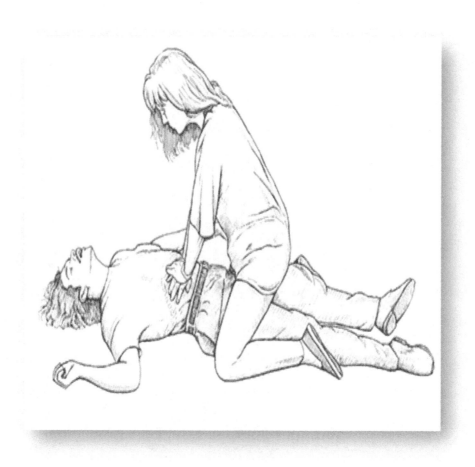

PART III

TAKING CARE OF YOURSELF

CHAPTER 29

---·<·>✦<·>·—

TAKE CARE OF YOURSELF
Sue Bell and Dr. Sally Burbank

Here is a sobering statistic: Thirty percent of caregivers die before the patient they are caring for does. Caretaking can age a person, so it is vital that you not neglect your own health. You cannot care for your loved one if you die first!

The good news? A lot of people have walked in your shoes, and because they have "been there, done that," they can offer a lot of practical advice. Here are some pearls of wisdom we gleaned from interviewing dozens of caregivers and nursing home staff:

Advice from Other Caregivers

• Get a thorough diagnosis so you will know the type of dementia you are facing, then research every source you can on the condition. Every situation is unique and should be treated as such. Not all dementias are Alzheimer's. Lewy body dementia and vascular dementia act differently than Alzheimer's disease.

• As the disease progresses, patients seem to focus on only one thing at a time, and that thing can change with time. If something doesn't work the first time, don't give up—it may work at a later stage.

• Help patients communicate. They get frustrated when they can't think of a word, and the more time they spend searching for the word, the more likely they are to forget their entire train of thought. Thus, if you think you know the word they are trying to come up with, fill in the blank. If it is not the correct word, ask them to describe what they are trying to say. For example, if the patient says, "That stuff you put on potatoes," you can offer, "Gravy?" Don't make the patient stumble around and try to come up with the word on her own, or she may get frustrated and sputter, "Oh, forget it." When you fill in the blank, you allow the patient to communicate for as long as possible. As the disease progresses, use hand gestures, pantomime, or point to pictures to communicate.

• If the patient accuses you of stealing something, deflect the accusation by saying something like, "I bet I misplaced it when I tidied up last night," or, "I'll see if I can find it later." Don't tell the patient in a patronizing tone, "Nobody stole the remote control, Ma. You probably lost it again." This can trigger a spat. Always remember to put yourself in the mindset of the patient and then try to alleviate their concerns.

• At family reunions, instruct people to avoid saying, "Do you know who I am?" It puts the patient on the spot, and she will likely feel obligated to lie and say, "Of course," even if she doesn't have a clue who the person is. Instead, ask people to introduce themselves (or, if it is easier, you do the introductions) with a gentle reminder of how they know the patient. For example, "Hi Grandpa, I'm your grandson, Erik. I'm a junior at Tennessee Tech this year." If the patient makes an insulted retort like, "I know who you are," have Erik reply, "Really? There are so many people here, I don't know how you keep track of us all," or, "People always confuse me with my brother, Mark, so I wanted you to know it was me," or, "I've grown an inch since the last time you saw me, so I wasn't sure you'd recognize me." This provides a face-saving out for the patient. Have family members come one at a time so the patient doesn't get overwhelmed. Name tags can help, also.

• Print up small business cards that read, "She has dementia. Thank you for understanding." If the patient is acting in a peculiar way in public, discretely hand the offended person a card. Most people, if they know why your loved one is acting strangely, will understand.

Caretaker: Care for Thyself!

With a potential span of over seven years from diagnosis to death, Alzheimer's caregiving is a marathon, not a sprint. You therefore need to take care of yourself, so you can maintain the stamina needed to make it through the long haul.

From the time I quit work to stay home full time to care for Ray, nine years passed before he died. There were days when I didn't think I could continue, but I had made a commitment to my husband and to myself that I would care for him. Somehow, God gave me the ability to do it one day at a time.

There is tremendous satisfaction in helping others. In the beginning, there were times when I got frustrated and had to force myself to be patient with Ray, but by the end of the day—because I had kept myself under control—I felt at peace.

As the disease progressed, Ray became easier to care for, more agreeable, and more cooperative. Ray was in the middle stage of AD when he was formally diagnosed. Sometimes I felt like the days would never end. I hired a woman to sit with Ray so that I could get out occasionally. In his last four months, we used Alive Hospice. I wish I had consulted them sooner.

An Eastern monarch once requested words of wisdom for when he went through difficult situations. He was given the phrase, "This too shall pass." Your patient will not survive this illness, so you will not be a caregiver forever.

Surprisingly, despite the hardships, I look back with fondness at our time together. Here are some additional suggestions that might help you:

Words of Advice

- **Take it one day, one hour, at a time.** It is less overwhelming that way. Jesus himself reminded us that one day's worry is enough for one day.

- **Get advice from others in your situation.** An online Facebook group for those who care for Alzheimer's patients can help you feel less isolated. The Alzheimer's Association is chocked full of useful information, and they can help you find a support group.

- **Take the path of least resistance.** Let the patient have his or her way as much as possible, unless it is unsafe. Pick your battles.

- **Take time for yourself**. Read. Go for walks. Play computer games. Garden.

- **Find a way to "have a life" every day.** As little as thirty minutes of "me" time can refresh you and prevent resentment.

- **Look for Alzheimer's daycares.** This will provide a reliable place to leave your loved one for a few hours, so you can attend appointments of your own or get a weekly break. Don't allow the patient to guilt-trip you out of bringing him to daycare just because he doesn't want to go. Often, he will have a good time once there, though he may not *remember* that from week to week. Because of his poor memory, he may act resistant each week, as though it were his first time. AD patients fear change and new caregivers. For you to remain a loving and patient caregiver, however, you *need* these breaks.

- **Watch funny movies or re-runs of "I love Lucy."** Laugh! Try to find things you can do with the patient that you both enjoy. Enjoy simple pleasures.

~ Remember: your physical and mental health are just as important as that of your loved one, so don't become a martyr who never gets out or has any fun. Don't neglect your own need for relaxation, exercise and companionship. If you behave like a martyr, your bad attitude will rub off onto your loved one. ~

How to Balance Your Needs with Your Loved One's

1. Solicit help. Family, friends, and church or synagogue members are often willing to help, but too many caregivers are hesitant to ask. Some caregivers resent that their friends and family don't intuitively see what's needed and volunteer. Newsflash: People cannot read your mind. You've got to *ask* for help, and you must *be specific* on what you need. For example, say, "I need someone to come stay with Ray for one hour on a Saturday morning once a month, so I can get a haircut. Could anyone in this Sunday school class help me with that?" Be specific and give plenty of notice so that people can put it in their schedules.

---

2. Hire a sitter or adult daycare once or twice a week. Three or four hours a week away from caregiving duties can do wonders for your mental health. When you get time for yourself, do things you enjoy like shopping, getting your hair or nails done, going for a massage, going for a long walk in the park, or working on your flower beds without interruption. Go to the library and read a good book or have lunch with a friend. Go for your dentist or doctor checkup.

3. Plan regular outings with friends and family. You mustn't allow yourself to become isolated and left out, or you will quickly become resentful and irritable. Bring your loved one to senior citizen luncheons to get out of the house.

From the beginning to the end of Ray's disease, our family went to a restaurant every week at a set time. This gave me something to look forward to. I got to see family and converse and laugh with others who were not memory challenged. The last time we met was one week before Ray died.

4. Don't balk at the money spent to hire a sitter. If the patient were in a nursing home, it would cost $226 a day. What you spend for a sitter once or twice a week is a pittance compared to that! Take out a reverse mortgage on your parent's house, if needed, to provide the funds for back-up caregivers.

To be at your best as a caregiver, you need to take care of yourself. You don't want to resent the time you spend taking care of your loved one. Figure out how to have a quality life *despite* the Alzheimer's. Yes, it can be a hassle to arrange for a sitter, but mental health breaks are crucial to avoid bitterness and burnout.

Caring for a family member with Alzheimer's is exhausting, so don't feel guilty about needing to get away. Just like when a baby is born, sleepless nights and chaos may reign until a new routine is established. With time, you will figure out how to balance your needs against those of your loved one.

5. Locate a reputable short-stay respite care facility in your area. There will come a time when you may need to go into the hospital for surgery, or go on a well-earned vacation, or attend your church's annual weekend retreat in a state park. Short-stay respite centers can provide the help needed to make this possible. They often have waiting lists, so make your plans well in advance.

Finding a place that is skilled in treating Alzheimer's patients can take digging, but the benefit of knowing you can get away for more than a few hours is important. You can search under short-stay residential care on Google, or better yet, call the Alzheimer's Association to see if they can suggest a reputable place near you. Their national phone number is 1(800) 272-3900.

6. Don't allow negative thoughts to fester. Dwelling on negative thoughts won't fix anything and will only spoil your outlook on life. You may then become impatient and rude toward the very person you want to help. Focus instead on what is good and positive in your life. Be thankful for all the modern conveniences and technology available to assist you. Treat yourself as you would treat your best friend if she were in this situation. You would encourage her, and if she made a mistake or had a hard day, you would remind her of the great care she provides most of the time. You would encourage her to get away regularly for mental health breaks.

7. Make sleep a priority. Sleep deprivation will make you grumpy and impatient. It will also weaken your immune system. If your patient is not sleeping well at night and is keeping you awake, sleep when you can, even if it means taking a nap in the afternoon. Also, set up activities around the house that the patient can do while you sleep at night. If you can keep your patient awake and entertained during the day, he will sleep better at night. Don't let him nod off in his chair throughout the day, or he won't sleep well at night.

Avoiding Depression

Depression is common in caregivers of AD patients for many reasons. The downward trajectory of your loved one's health is depressing, and the workload is exhausting and isolating. Plus, you have changed from being your spouse's lover to your spouse's nurse.

To combat depression, try some of the following:

Exercise regularly and maintain friendships. Aerobic exercise, such as walking, biking, or using exercise equipment, raises endorphins which are natural mood elevators. Stay in touch with family and friends, as isolation will aggravate your gray mood. Join an AD caregiver's group to gain mutual support and understanding. If there isn't one in your town, consider starting one. Check out the Alzheimer's Association Facebook page. In order to make connections with people who understand what you are going through, befriend them on Facebook.

If you can't leave the house much, connect with your friends on Facebook. I had two daughters and four siblings who lived close by, so I made a point of walking with one of them each morning. Ray and I went to lunch with three of my siblings every Thursday, and the laughter, adult conversation, and support became an anchor during the long years of being a full-time caregiver.

Keep your sense of humor. Watch funny movies or television programs. Read lighthearted books and jokes. Incorporate fun activities, holiday decorations, or themes, like wearing green on St. Patrick's Day or celebrating September 13—National Peanut Day—by eating peanut butter sandwiches and cookies.

Create ways of having fun. Even if you are stuck at home most of the time, you can host a pajama party, cook popcorn, put on colorful socks or slippers and festive pajamas, and watch a favorite movie together. Invite the grandkids or a friend to join you.

Invite friends over and ask them to wear a T-shirt from a special vacation spot. Have them bring photos of their trip to share. It needn't be a fancy meal; just call out for pizza. The point is to have fun and be around friends. Don't worry if the house isn't spick and span—your real friends know what you are going through and won't judge.

Watch a ballgame and pretend you are at the ballpark. Put on ball caps, cook hot dogs, drink colas, and create a wave every time your team scores. If you write these events on the calendar, these activities will give you something to look forward to and make your days more enjoyable.

Take a vacation vicariously. Check out a DVD from the library that features a specific country you have always wanted to visit. Pull out an atlas and locate the various cities and attractions mentioned in the film. Create a meal that features the cuisine of that country.

Invite another patient with AD and her caregiver over for a party. Serve fancy cookies and tea using a colorful teapot and teacups. (Not an expensive family heirloom, however!) Guests could also have fun wearing fancy Easter hats, as well.

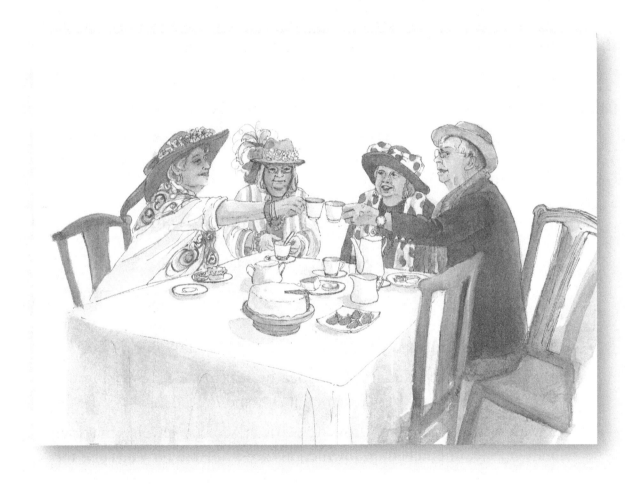

One caregiver I know celebrated Mozart's birthday every year, because her husband, who had AD, was a lifetime Mozart aficionado. They celebrated the special day by listening to Mozart symphonies and the Marriage of Figaro. They wore party hats and feasted on a cake decorated with musical notes. Her husband helped make the cake and frost it. A similar party could be planned around your loved one's favorite sports figure by wearing team T-shirts with the athlete's name and watching an old game. Bake a cake and frost it to look like a baseball or football field.

~ Believe it or not, this time of caregiving may give you an opportunity to enrich your life. You are somewhat housebound, and your days have slowed down, so you can take more time to do things you enjoy but haven't had time to do in the past. ~

With technology and social media, it is easy to stay connected with extended family and friends thanks to Facebook, Twitter, Snapchat, and Pinterest.

You need to stay positive because AD patients absorb good feelings like a sponge. Like children, they enjoy fun and living in the moment. Here are some additional things you can do:

More Ways to Take Care of Yourself:

- Catch up with friends through letters, phone calls or visits.

- Write letters to your grandchildren. Tell them how much they mean to you.

- Learn a foreign language through Duolingo or Rosetta Stone.

- Participate in a new exercise, like yoga or Jazzercize by checking out DVDs from the library so you can do it at home.

- Take up writing, painting, growing African violets, jewelry making, woodworking, or crocheting. Instructions are available on YouTube for almost anything. These are activities that can be done in small snippets of time. Devoting just fifteen minutes a day to an activity will eventually lead to some level of competence.

- Research your family's genealogy through computer sites like Ancestry.com.

- Try something new. Take up a musical instrument or learn to draw. Make yourself do it!

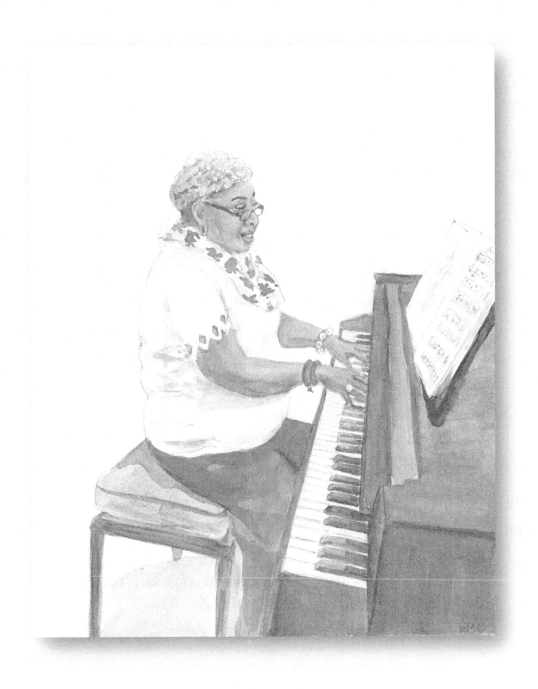

- Play computer games like "Words with Friends" with family members, friends, or even complete strangers.

- Skype with friends or relatives who live far away.

- Start a card game or Yahtzee club that meets in your home. You can have the AD patient look over your shoulder and be your "partner." You can let your loved one roll the dice or hold the cards while you make the decisions.

~ Consider this period of your life a gift of time. When daily tasks become cumbersome, remember the saying, "Whistle while you work." ~

- When brushing your patient's hair, sing their favorite song.

- When brushing their teeth, hum a happy tune or favorite hymn.

- When helping your spouse dress, quote a favorite Scripture.

- When doing housework and laundry, play uplifting music. (Classical music seems to help keep patients calm. CDs are available from the library. Consider listening to famous works of the major composers.)

- Make up dance steps to the patient's favorite music. It's okay if you look ridiculous. Who's watching? Just live in the moment and have fun! Plus, it will give you some exercise.

In short, make an intentional effort to look at the positive aspects of your situation. Use this time constructively. As Sally's mother loves to remind her:

**~ When you can't change your circumstances,
change your attitude! ~**

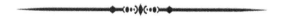

CHAPTER 30

———◆••◦••〉◆〈••◦••◆———

SUPPORT GROUPS FOR CAREGIVERS
Dr. Sally Burbank

One of the best things a caregiver can do to avoid isolation is to find other caregivers in the community who are taking care of their loved ones with dementia. Start by contacting your local Alzheimer's Association to see if they know of an existing support group you could join. Their national toll-free phone number is (800) 272-3900. Or check with assisted living facilities, senior citizen centers, or even Alive Hospice.

If no support group exists, start your own by notifying churches in your town that you are starting one. Meetings can be weekly or monthly, but the main goal is to make connections with other caregivers to offer mutual support and advice. Once you have made the connections, you have a friend to lean on.

If anyone in the group has a large living room and likes to entertain, the group could meet in her home. Or if you want to avoid the added workload of anyone having to clean the house or make refreshments before meetings, you could meet at a neutral location like a church, restaurant, assisted living center conference room, or a senior citizen center. Perhaps the support group could meet in a separate room while the patients eat lunch at the senior citizens center every Wednesday, for example. Caregivers could take turns stepping out of the meeting to assist patients with eating. Or better yet? Hire someone for an hour to oversee the patients and then split the cost amongst the group.

Some groups bring cupcakes and party hats to celebrate the birthdays that occur that month, and everyone sings, "Happy Birthday." Perhaps the "birthday boys and girls" could bring photos from their childhood or young adult years to share.

Potluck dinners for patients and caregivers could be planned monthly with disposable plates and cups for easy cleanup. Make it fun by selecting a theme. Here are some possibilities:

Possible Monthly Party Themes

January: Silly Socks and Hat Day. Everyone dons silly duds to make it fun.

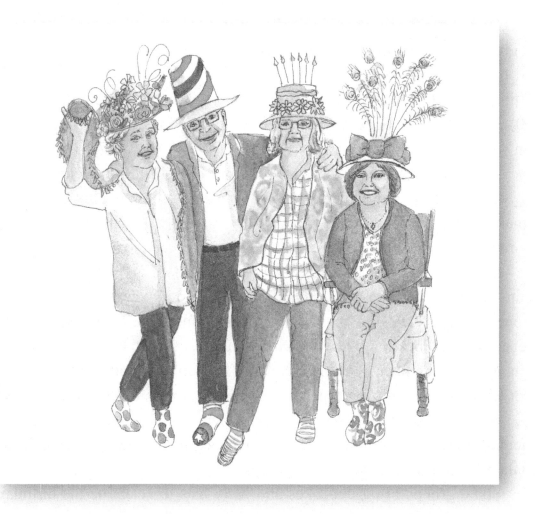

February: Valentine's Day. AD patients could design simple Valentines from construction paper and doilies to give to someone. Serve heart-shaped cookies. Ask patients and caregivers to share how they met their spouse, fell in love, where they honeymooned, etc. If single, ask if she ever had a beau.

March: St. Patrick's Day. Everyone wears green. Add green food coloring to ginger ale or water. Serve cupcakes with green frosting.

April: Women wear something with a flower—either a dress, blouse, brooch, or scarf. Men wear a gardening straw cap or overalls. Decorate the house with a colorful bouquet of flowers. Attendees could color pictures of flowers.

May: In honor of Mother's Day, everyone brings pictures of their mothers, sisters, and daughters to share and discuss. What was your mother like? (Or stepmother, aunt, or daughter.) What were your mother's favorite sayings?

June: In honor of Father's Day, everyone brings pictures of their fathers, brothers, and sons to share and discuss. What do you remember about your father (or step-father or uncle/grandfather)? What was his best advice?

July: Wear red, white, and blue. Cut up strawberries and blueberries and serve with whipped cream. Give everyone a small flag to wave as you sing "America the Beautiful" or color an American flag.

August: Play a DVD showing America's national parks in the background with the sound turned off while everyone talks about their favorite vacation spots. Caregivers could bring pictures to pass around.

September: School Days. Have everyone bring an old yearbook or classroom picture. Laugh at the hairstyles and reminisce about what they remember about school. What was their favorite subject? Least favorite? Who did they have a crush on? Since Alzheimer's patients often retain their old memories until late stage, this is a fun one!

October: Halloween. Everyone wears orange or Fall-themed clothing, or, if they want, a costume. Provide pumpkins to decorate with magic markers. Serve pumpkin pie or pumpkin bread. If colorful deciduous trees are in your area, bring in pretty leaves for patients to examine. Let each patient select a maple/gingko leaf and then turn it into a coaster by ironing it between pieces of waxed paper.

November: Thanksgiving/Harvest. Serve vegetable soup and turkey slices and ask if anyone ever lived or worked on a farm. If so, tell what it was like. Ask everyone to share what they are thankful for.

December: Christmas. Everyone comes dressed in Christmas colors (or Hanukkah colors, if Jewish) or silly sweaters. Sing easy Christmas carols, and bring decorated cookies or goodies. Or, better yet, participants could decorate their own cookies at the party with colored sugar and sprinkles. Sugar cookie dough can be purchased in a roll ready to bake.

Other monthly themes could include: "Wear your favorite dress or shirt," or "Wear your favorite scarf/brooch/necklace or necktie," or "Wear a ball cap or T-shirt of your favorite sports team." Theme-based parties offer a festive but simple way to give patients and caregivers something to look forward to. Planning should not become a hassle for the caregiver and should only utilize clothes, photos, or other items lying around the house.

Many advanced AD patients won't understand what is going on at the party, but they will absorb the smiles, laughter, and fun around them, and they will enjoy the snacks and visual stimuli. Even patients with advanced AD pick up on a happy vibe in a room.

~ Theme-based parties are as beneficial to caregivers as they are to patients. ~

The parties give you an excuse to meet with friends, to do something fun, and to have something to look forward to. Since these parties allow mild and moderate-stage AD patients to reminisce about the past, most patients enjoy them. If the caregivers register excitement, it will usually trickle down to the patients. If your loved one resists going to a party, don't rise to the bait. Inform her calmly that you are going because it would be rude to back out at the last minute, and that it is good for both of you to get out and socialize.

~ If your loved one is a killjoy about going to social events, don't give advanced notice, or she may fret and refuse to go. Only you, the caregiver, need to know the plan in advance. ~

Don't let planning parties become overwhelming: meetings can go back to simple get-togethers. Reassure caregivers that it is okay to bring their loved one in a bathrobe and slippers on the day of the party if their patient is being ornery and won't cooperate. The get-togethers should not create a power struggle of having to get the patient bathed and dressed in fancy clothes against their will. Everyone in the group will understand if your loved one shows up looking bedraggled, if that is the best you can do. (Now if *you* show up in a torn bathrobe…)

A closed Facebook group should be established for all caregivers in the group to provide support between meetings. If needed, ask your child or grandchild to assist you in setting it up. Double check first to see if one already exists by calling the local Alzheimer's Association.

Friendships with other caregivers will naturally develop, and you will quickly discover which Alzheimer's patients seem to get along. Perhaps you could arrange weekly caregiving exchanges. You could offer to take your new friend's mother on a Thursday afternoon drive and stop for ice cream along the way in exchange for your new friend watching your mother every Tuesday afternoon. This will allow each of you a guaranteed break every week free-of-charge. Plus, it really is no more work to take two AD patients for an afternoon drive than one. Just make sure both patients have gone to the bathroom immediately before you leave, and that both have on clean, disposable underwear.

Entertaining two AD patients can include a trip to the park to watch children play or going to a dog park to watch the dogs. Bring a picnic basket with cut up fruit and cookies or eat lunch at a mom-and-pop diner. If the patients can still walk, a trip to an old cemetery to look at tombstones can be fun.

If it is raining or cold, color pretty pictures in adult coloring books, work a simple jigsaw puzzle, play Yahtzee, Bingo, or Crazy Eights. You will need to guide them, but remember, it doesn't matter if they botch up the rules—the goal is to have fun. As the AD advances, simplify the rules to just shaking until all five dice are 1's, then 2's, then 3's and so on.

Planet Earth DVDs, with their beautiful photography from around the world, can be enjoyable, as can looking at coffee table books of America's national parks, or scenic places from around the world. Check out a book of famous paintings from the library and look at it together. Ask them which paintings they like best. Look at old photo albums, and if the patients are still in the early-to-middle stage, talk about their childhoods.

Roll out sugar cookies and have the patients use cookie cutters and then frost and decorate the cookies after they are baked.

Rules for Successful Support Group Meetings

The goal of support groups is not just to have fun parties. The real purpose is to provide a safe place for caregivers to share the cornucopia of emotions that caring for a loved one with AD triggers. Nothing bolsters a caregiver more than knowing her feelings—not all nice—are common. Meetings should motivate caregivers to open up and share feelings and provide a place to solve problems and exchange ideas, such as, "Here's what worked for me when my Mom did that ..."

Set ground rules and distribute them in writing. They should include:

- **No gossiping.** What is said in the group stays in the group, unless the member specifically gives permission to share what she said. Why? Members will feel betrayed if their feelings are exposed, even if disguised as, "Pray for Margie because she said ..." This is still betraying the confidence of a group member, and she will shut down and never open up again if she doesn't think her words are kept confidential. If you want your prayer group to pray for Margie, get Margie's permission first.

- **No monopolizing the conversation.** In any group, some members are more talkative than others, which is fine. A motormouth, who dominates the entire meeting and doesn't allow others to get a word in edgewise, is not! It will frustrate the other members and lead to resentment and poor attendance. If it becomes necessary, you can use a tennis ball that is handed from one member to another, and no one is allowed to talk until they are holding the ball. If one member talks too long, you can set a timer for five minutes, and when the timer goes off, let her know it is time to give someone else a chance to speak. The leader needs to take control and not be afraid to say something like, "Phyllis, thank you for sharing. Let's open the floor so everyone gets an equal opportunity to talk. Who else would like to share this morning?"

- **No shaming.** Remind group members there are no "wrong" feelings, only wrong behaviors. Caretaking patients with AD can sometimes trigger a host of negative emotions: anger, hurt, frustration, exasperation, shame, guilt, grief, and resentment. On a bad day, a caregiver will wish her husband (or mother) with AD would hurry up and die, but then feel guilty about having such thoughts. Members must feel safe to share these feelings without a fellow member piping in, "That's terrible," or, "You shouldn't feel that way," or some version of, "Buck up!"

- **No know-it-alls.** One of the goals of the support group is to learn from each other. Having a "know-it-all", who trivializes problems or acts like she has all the answers, can intimidate members and make them feel inadequate. Stress that the best way to share advice is to say something like, "This may not work for everyone, but here is what worked for me ..."

Sample Questions to Ask at Meetings:

- What is the biggest challenge you are facing right now?
- What do you need to do to take better care of your own needs?
- What would most help you in your caregiver role?
- What can you do to get the help you need? Who can you ask for help? Who can you hire?

- What services are available in our area? Senior citizen daycares? Senior citizen lunches? Where can I bring Mom if I want to get away for the weekend with my husband? What about a week's vacation?

- How do I handle my resentment that my sister doesn't help more, or that my father is never grateful for anything I do for him?

- How can I balance Mom's needs with those of my husband and kids? I feel like I'm failing everyone.

- How can I fit exercise and "me" time into my schedule? I am exhausted!

- I hate being a caregiver! I never wanted to be somebody's nurse, but there's no one else to do it. How can I change my attitude?

- How can I stay positive when my mother stays so irritable and negative?

- My father never wants to leave the house, but I feel trapped and resentful. Do I make him go against his will? I feel guilty when I make him do things he doesn't want to do.

- At this stage of Mother's AD, how long can I safely leave her alone? Can I be gone an hour to run to the grocery store?

- Mom doesn't have the money for assisted living, but she doesn't need to be living alone any more. What are my options?

- Mom refuses to leave her home, but she's no longer safe to stay alone. What do I do?

- I'm not sure Dad should be driving any more. He hit the mailbox backing out but insists he is still fit to drive. He mostly goes to the grocery store and church. I would hate to be responsible for all his transportation, but I don't want him to get into an accident. Who can competently and objectively evaluate his driving skills? How do I make him give up the car keys if he's not fit to drive anymore?

CHAPTER 31

HOW CHURCHES AND FAMILY CAN HELP
Dr. Sally Burbank

If I could suggest one thing churches (or synagogues or Senior Citizen Centers) could do to benefit caregivers, it would be to provide a once-a-week drop-off adult daycare to free up caregivers for a few hours each week to run necessary errands. Caregivers could bring their loved one at noon with a simple brown bag lunch and return at three.

Be sure to check the size limits and licensing requirements for your state. In Tennessee, for example, the regulations start when you have ten or more individuals for more than three hours. Thus, if you kept it to nine or fewer patients for three hours maximum, you would not be considered a licensed adult daycare and could by-pass all the red tape. You need at least two caregivers and access to a handicapped bathroom.

Activities could include Bingo, coloring, a large-piece jigsaw puzzle, simple craft projects, Planet Earth videos, and sing-a-longs. Some AD patients enjoy games such as tossing a beanbag into a bucket (which can be done even in a wheelchair). Patients in the later stages may spend most of their time just sitting and observing, but this is okay since they often enjoy watching the activity. A snack of cookies or goldfish could break up the activities. Small prizes for Bingo winners are popular.

Since AD patients have poor short-term memories, the activities can be repeated week to week. Caregivers quickly learn which activities patients like and which are a flop.

Sometimes the support group itself can run the daycare, with each caregiver committing to stay with the patients one week in exchange for three weeks off. Or, caregivers could rotate hourly so that each gets to attend two hours of the support group. Helpers could also be hired, as long as they are dependable and patient.

The daycare should have no less than one adult for every five patients, depending on the severity and challenges of the participants. There should always be at least two caregivers present, as a patient could wander off in the time it takes to bring a patient to the bathroom. Hired caregivers would need some training in how to work with AD patients. (Give them a copy of the Caregiver Pearls.)

Here is some additional advice for a successful daycare experience:

Never ask a patient if he *wants* to go to daycare or Senior Citizens. I guarantee for many the answer will be an automatic, "No!" Alzheimer's patients often reject social interactions, even if they had a great time the previous week. Why? They don't *remember* having a good time, so to them it is a frightening, new experience.

Don't make it a choice. Don't ask if he wants to go, and don't give him advanced notice that he is going, or he may balk from the minute you mention it until you arrive at the daycare. Giving advance notice just agitates patients and adds unnecessary stress. Don't be held hostage by the patient's anxiety. As long as you know the patient will receive loving and sufficient care, go! Too many caregivers give their loved one a choice about attending groups, and their lives end up being controlled by the patient's negative and fearful attitude.

Instead, tell your loved one you are going for a ride. Leave a few minutes early and point out houses you like along the way so that you are not lying to him. When you reach the daycare or Senior Citizen's Center say, "We're going to go in and get a snack together."

Stay calm, positive, and pleasant, no matter how negative or argumentative Dad becomes. Act excited about where you are going and try to distract him from his negativity by talking about what kind of snack the center will serve today. Don't argue or debate whether to go inside or not, or you will give the patient control.

Remember, you are the one with a fully functioning brain, not the patient. It isn't good for either of you to sit in the house, isolated and watching television all day long. As the caregiver, you must take the reins and make the patient get out and socialize whether he wants to or not! Why?

~ Staying social helps slow the progression of AD. Going to a daycare or Senior Citizen Center is for the patient's own good! ~

If you act excited about going, the patient will register your enthusiasm and feel less afraid. Once inside, offer your loved one a treat and stay until he is situated and busy with something like Bingo or a jigsaw puzzle.

If a patient refuses to get out of the car, don't argue. Simply pick up his feet, swivel them out of the car, and then lift the patient into a standing position.

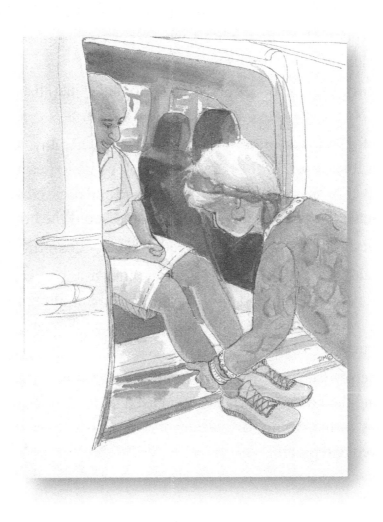

The first time you go to a daycare, stay with the patient for at least thirty minutes until he gets comfortable. You can then say you have to run a few errands and will return soon. Plan to be gone for only an hour or so the first few visits.

If the patient frets about you leaving, leave a large construction paper clock with the hands pointing to the hour you will return. Be sure he is participating in an activity when you leave.

How Friends and Family Can Support Caregivers
Sue Bell

1. **Call and let the caregiver know you are thinking of them.** When I felt like no one else knew what I was experiencing, a phone call was such a welcome relief. *Someone cares!*

2. **Let the caregiver talk.** If they want to talk, just listen and don't interrupt. No advice is needed unless they ask for it.

3. **Drop by for an occasional visit** and bring a healthy, easy-to-chew casserole. It is easier for the caregiver if you come to her house than for the caregiver to have to get the patient bathed and dressed to go to yours. Wear casual clothes so she won't be embarrassed if the house is a mess.

4. **Bake something** like homemade bread or a tasty dessert.

5. **Offer to take the patient for a joy ride** so the caregiver can get a break. Patients love to ride around and stop for ice cream along the way. This is an easy way to entertain a patient, and it frees the caregiver up for a couple hours.

6. **Offer to help with yard work or small maintenance**—Assist with odd jobs around the house that the husband used to do. Things like changing light bulbs in the ceiling or putting on winter tires pose problems for overworked caregivers.

7. **Offer to sit with a patient for a day**, or better yet, a weekend, so the caregiver can celebrate a birthday with a much-needed weekend retreat.

8. **Donate an hour every other week to housecleaning tasks.** Offer to help change the bedsheets, vacuum, mop the kitchen floor—tasks that the caregiver may procrastinate doing because they are strenuous or tiresome. This can be presented as a birthday or Christmas gift if you are afraid of offending the caregiver by suggesting she needs a housekeeper.

After the Patient Dies

1. **Watch what you say.** Don't make comments like, "He's better off now because he isn't suffering anymore." The patient wasn't really aware he was suffering, and the caregiver is feeling conflicting emotions. Platitudes don't help. It's okay if the caregiver says this, but not you!

2. **Don't be afraid to mention the deceased person's name.** Relate something positive about the person, such as a cherished memory.

3. **Look for ways to help the person who is left behind.** In my case, I needed help with trimming the shrubs and home repairs. A thoughtful neighbor, sons-in-law, and grandchildren stepped in to help.

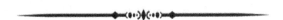

CHAPTER 32

—◆‹••›◗‹••›◆—

END OF LIFE DECISIONS
Sue Bell and Dr. Sally Burbank

The patient's wishes for end-of-life treatment should be thoroughly discussed and legal documents signed when the patient is first diagnosed. By the middle and late stages, cognitive ability is so compromised she may not comprehend well enough to make sound decisions.

The following forms need to be filled out and signed as soon after the diagnosis as possible:

- Wills
- Living Wills
- No Code/DRN orders
- Powers of attorney (Legal, financial, medical)

Funeral and burial decisions should also be discussed—cremation versus coffin, cemetery plot, what to inscribe on the tombstone, favorite hymns for the memorial service, etc. Ask these questions sooner rather than later. Also, since coffins and funerals are expensive, be sure the patient has the money or life insurance to cover burial expenses.

Final Days

The end of life is probably the most difficult time for the family and caregiver. After a long struggle, battle fatigue is at an all-time high. You have already lost your loved one mentally and emotionally, and now you are losing them physically. There is only a shell of the person you once knew and loved left. All you can do now is keep him comfortable. Don't be afraid to express your feelings; reach out and ask for help.

In his final days, my goal was to keep Ray comfortable with palliative care. I did not want to prolong his life since I knew Ray did not want extreme measures taken. Organizations such as Alive Hospice can help tremendously with this. Enlist their help when the doctor thinks your loved one's longevity is six months or less.

Your loved one's doctor can assist you on what is appropriate. CPR and feeding tubes are no longer recommended in end-stage AD. In fact, after an exhaustive review of all available studies, The American Geriatric Society released a position paper in 2014 strongly *discouraging* the use of feeding tubes at all in AD patients. This is also the position of the Alzheimer's Association.

Why? Surprisingly, feeding tubes were *not* found to prolong life or reduce the risk for aspirating food into the lungs. Instead, they were shown to *increase* the following:

Feeding tubes increase the following:

- **Agitation**. Patients can become fixated on trying to pull out their tube.

- **Aspiration**. Patients often reflux the liquid tube feed out of their stomach and into their lungs, which can lead to aspiration pneumonia.

- **Bedsores**. By prolonging the length of time that a patient lies in bed (thin and largely immobile), the risk of bedsores increases exponentially. Because patients try to pull out their feeding tubes, they are often kept in restraints or doped up in nursing homes. This leaves them lying on their back day and night, which causes excessive pressure on delicate skin of the back and hip area. Deep bedsores are often the end result.

- **Trauma**. Patients may traumatize their stomachs when they tug on or yank out their feeding tube. A tear or hole in the stomach is a surgical emergency.

- **Expense.** Tube-feeding is expensive and offers no extra quality of life to justify the cost.

"But," you may ask, "How can I let Mama starve to death? Won't she be hungry and thirsty?"

Thankfully, when AD patients reach the point they can no longer eat, they do not feel hungry and typically do *not* want to eat. In fact, it just seems to annoy them when family members badger them constantly to eat.

Weight loss is the natural progression of the disease, so the caregiver should not feel guilty about it. There is no cure for AD, and studies document that life is not prolonged with tube-feeding.

~Careful hand-feeding of soft foods with the patient sitting up fully is the preferred way to nourish patients~

Hand-feeding patients can take twenty to thirty minutes per meal because AD patients are very slow eaters. Truthfully, the reason nursing homes resorted to feeding tubes is because hand-feeding every late-stage Alzheimer's patient at every meal became too labor intensive: they simply didn't have the staff to spend thirty minutes with every patient.

By the last week of life, the patient will sleep most of the time—up to twenty hours a day. Not eating or drinking is nature's way of allowing Alzheimer's patients to die peacefully in their sleep. Without supplemental fluids, the kidneys gradually shut down, and the patient goes into a coma and dies without suffering.

CHAPTER 33

GRIEF AND LEARNING TO MOVE ON
Sue Bell

"Grief never ends—but it changes. It's a passage, not a place to stay. Grief is not a sign of weakness nor a lack of faith: It is the price of love."

Ray died on August 20, 2013. He handled his journey with Alzheimer's with more grace and joy than I could ever have imagined.

During our fifty-three years of marriage, we were a team. After his death, I missed the security of having a partner, and some days I felt completely lost without him. Initially, I felt I had lost my whole world, and I wasn't sure how to go on. I had dedicated nine long years to caring for him. In his honor, however, I looked for ways to cope and find meaning in my life without him.

Finding a new normal can be difficult. My days while Ray was alive revolved predominantly around caring for him. Suddenly that role was gone. I now had complete freedom, but I found myself not wanting to go anywhere, do anything or see anyone. When I went out in public, people asked how I was doing, and I'd tear up or break down sobbing. Talk about embarrassing. Then doubts flooded me. Had I done everything I could have for Ray? Did I handle things the right way? Memories of when I had been impatient flooded over me. Flashbacks of seemingly insignificant events or conversations surfaced, and I found myself reliving those moments and reviewing my life. My grieving and self-reflection went on for weeks. I have since learned this is all part of the healing process.

Thankfully, with time, I began to experience moments of peace and joy again. I knew I had a choice: I could become reclusive and bitter, or I could become better. I chose the latter. I would cherish all the good memories of my life with Ray and put away the memories that caused me pain. I would embrace good times with friends and family again.

Yes, stabbing memories still surfaced. Unwelcomed memories would pop up out of nowhere, and the next thing I knew, I would be sobbing when five minutes earlier I had been perfectly fine. This, too, is normal. Holidays, birthdays, anniversaries, and family events were especially difficult.

Grieving takes time. In the olden days, widows wore black for a year to signify they were in mourning. The black clothes helped alert others that the widow might become weepy or reclusive after the loss of a spouse. Today, people often don't allow enough time to recover from a major loss before jumping into something new.

Many widows struggle with indecision after their husband dies. Do I sell the house and move into a condo? What about assisted living? Do I get rid of his stuff, so it doesn't trigger me? Do I go to events we always went to as a couple, or will it be too painful? Do I consider going out with that nice widower at church who has shown an interest in me?

Most geriatric specialists recommend not making ANY major life decisions, such as selling a house or remarrying, for a full year after the spouse's death, since major decisions made when emotions are volatile and raw often lead to regret. It is fine to make needed improvements in the house that may have been put off due to the stress of caregiving, but don't sell your home outright until emotions have settled down.

Too often I have seen widows sell their lifelong home after their husband dies out of fear or impulse or pressure from their children. Later on, they bitterly regret losing their beloved flower beds or sunroom or privacy. Remember, yardwork and home repairs can be hired out. Also, moving to a new place will not make the memories of your life in the old home magically disappear. If the widow's health is good, she should not feel pressured to sell her home or move into a condo/assisted living until she is emotionally stable and convinced it is the right decision.

Some widows feel anxious being alone at night for the first time, and many have trouble sleeping. I encourage these women to thoroughly lock up the house, keep a charged cellphone next to the bed, and have ambient noise (a fan, soft music, or the sound of waves on a DVD) playing in the bedroom to drown out the noise of the house creaking.

People experience a wide range of emotions after losing a loved one to AD, including guilt, anger, frustration, relief, indecision, freedom, anxiety, deep sorrow, self-pity, and depression. You may experience any or all of these emotions, and they may change from one minute to the next.

Mary M. felt so worn-out from eight years of caring for her mother that she'd often wished her mother would hurry up and die. When her mother finally did die, she felt guilty for having had those thoughts. She didn't really want to lose her mother; she just couldn't stand seeing her progressively dwindle. Plus, she was exhausted from all the work. Mary is not alone. Conflicting emotions are perfectly normal.

You will probably feel a sense of relief that the ordeal is over. You can finally get a good night of sleep and have your freedom back. You may then feel like a heel for being relieved your loved one is dead. Ten minutes later, you may become depressed and teary that you've lost him. You may feel angry that you devotedly took care of your husband, but he won't be around to take care of you. You may resent that he died and left you all alone. You may wish you had died with him. All of these feelings are normal because feelings don't have to be rational—they just are.

The current belief is that grief has five stages, though it is not necessary to experience all five, and the stages may not always occur in an exact order. Some phases last longer than others, and sometimes people go through two or more stages simultaneously. The family of an Alzheimer's patient experiences the grief process three times: when first diagnosed, when witnessing the patient's progressive decline, (especially when they no longer know who you are), and when the patient dies. The grief process for a caregiver usually involves these stages:

Stages of Grief

1. Denial
2. Anger
3. Bargaining with God
4. Depression
5. Acceptance

Once you catch up on your sleep and feel ready to forge ahead with life, evaluate the course you want to take. Ask yourself, "What is it I have always wanted to do but couldn't because I was caretaking? There are many choices:

What Do I Do Now?

Ideas for moving on with life after the death of your loved one.

- Travel.
- Learn to play the piano.
- Learn a foreign language.
- Volunteer at a school, hospital, or nursing home.
- Visit homebound people.
- Bake a pie or cake for someone who has little or no family.
- Clean out and unload all the junk from your messy closets.
- Attend your grandchildren's sporting events and take them out to eat.
- Meet a friend for lunch.
- Browse through antique stores.
- Plant a flower garden.
- Go to lectures, concerts and art museums.
- Become a foster grandparent.
- Volunteer at the church nursery or Sunday school. (Babies and little ones will help you focus on life and vitality again.)
- Volunteer one day a week at an adult daycare for Alzheimer's patients.

- Create new traditions around the holidays by decorating differently.
- Change the paint colors in your house or redecorate.
- Sign up for a knitting or crocheting class.
- Take an exercise or water aerobics class.

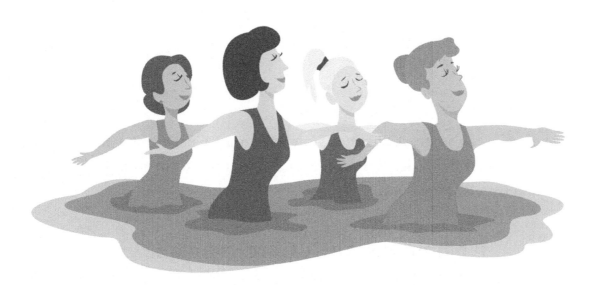

New beginnings may be uncomfortable at first, but they can be healing, and they make a statement that you are moving forward with life.

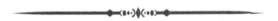

CHAPTER 34

A GLIMPSE INSIDE A MEMORY CARE CENTER

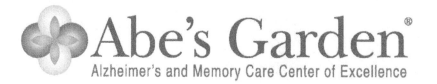

Abe's Garden is an Alzheimer's and Memory Care Center in Nashville, Tennessee. It opened its doors in 2015 and currently serves forty-two live-in residents and twenty outpatients.

What makes Abe's Garden unique?

Abe's Garden provides care that is evidence-based and person-centered. Its many enrichment activities and family interactions are performed by a trained and supportive staff. It is the first memory care center in the country to be a site of ongoing research and teaching, thereby setting standards for memory care treatment centers around the world.

Person-centered care means focusing on what the patient can still *do*, rather than on lost abilities. Abe's Garden provides a wide variety of engaging activities appropriate to the patient's stage of dementia, such as tai chi, pet therapy, photography, flower arranging, choir, drum circle, and community service projects. Additionally, members and caregivers receive emotional support as they build relationships with others in a similar situation.

Activities of daily living—such as eating, bathing, and sleeping—occur according to the individual patient's preferences, not by a predetermined schedule.

Abe's Garden, with the help of the Vanderbilt Center for Quality Aging, continually assesses the effectiveness of their programs and makes improvements. The research findings are then shared to caregivers throughout the nation using a series of short, informational videos. Video topics include communication, dealing with reactive behavior, mouth care, bathing and dressing assistance, one-on-one engagement, using music to engage, exercise, end of life planning, and talking to children about Alzheimer's. These videos are available free-of-charge via **abesgarden.org** or the Abe's Garden YouTube channel. Check them out!

I recently interviewed the staff at Abe's Garden via a written questionnaire to get their perspective on caretaking Alzheimer's patients. Here are some of their responses:

QUESTIONS & ANSWERS from ABE'S GARDEN

1. Caregivers are often plagued with guilt when circumstances demand admitting their loved one to a nursing home or memory care center. What reassurance can you provide to guilt-ridden caregivers? What are the advantages of living in a community like Abe's Garden?

JUDY GIVEN, *Director of Campus Development:*

Being a caregiver can be exhausting, and often caregivers put their own needs last. As a result, it's common for the caregiver to pass away first. I advise caregivers to approach their situation as flight attendants advise travelers on airplanes: "Put your oxygen mask on first, so you can better assist others."

When I work with a family that is struggling with the decision to transition their loved one to a senior living community, I acknowledge the weight of the commitments and promises they may have previously made regarding their loved one's care. I then reframe this commitment as not being one they must shoulder alone. Identifying and selecting an optimal care environment, with trained staff to meet their loved one's needs, is also caring for someone "in sickness and in health." People age differently, and an AD patient's needs don't always allow them to stay in a home environment, especially if the health of the caregiver is jeopardized.

BRENDA NAGEY, *Director of Life Engagement:*

At Abe's Garden, those with dementia benefit from the structured stimulation that surpasses what is available in most homes. We absorb much of the caregiving responsibilities so that family members may simply enjoy *being* with their loved one. During visits, my colleagues and I encourage families to participate with their loved one in our programs. This way, they can witness firsthand how we successfully communicate with patients, such as asking questions that provide simple choices and are failure-free to answer.

BEVERLY THEIS, *Licensed Social Worker:*

Providing care 24/7 can lead to caregiver stress and burnout, as the role can become all-consuming. Memory care communities like Abe's Garden offer disease-appropriate engagement, quality caregiving, emotional support, and medication management. It's not giving up, it's *enhancing* their loved one's quality of life.

2.   What can smooth the transition from living at home to living in a memory care community, assisted living facility, or nursing home?

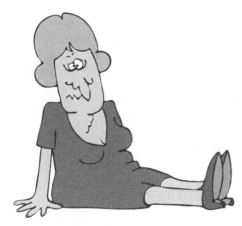

JUDY GIVEN, *Director of Campus Development:*

The steps to a smooth transition are different for each individual. I recommend families visit memory-care centers long before a loved one needs to leave home. This provides the opportunity to identify preferences before things reach a critical stage. Also, I recommend getting on waiting lists for preferred communities so if the need for a transition suddenly arises, the family will have one or more options.

People with memory issues may not recall the discussions about their new home, so they often benefit from eating lunch with those already living in the memory care community a few times before the move. Abe's Garden has a day program called The Club, which allows non-residents to experience the program before moving in, which eases the anxiety.

3. What should the caregiver say or do if the patient hates living in the nursing home or memory-care community and insists he wants to go home? How should the caregiver handle the guilt-trip a patient dishes out?

BEVERLY THEIS, *Licensed Social Worker:*

I suggest speaking with the resident about what he is thinking about when he says "home." The answer may not be what you anticipate. Sometimes the individual simply wants to feel more comfortable, sometimes they are in pain or upset. I recommend replying with, "Tell me about your home. What are you thinking about?"

Give the resident approximately three months to adjust to the transition.

Ask advice from the staff about recommended times of day to visit, how often to visit, and suggested activities during visits. It's often helpful for family members to join the resident in the engagement activities at the memory-care center. Become a part of the patient's new world by joining her in Bingo or crafts.

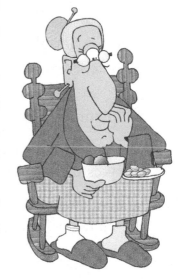

The family member's reaction is extremely important in each phase of the transition process. If the family member does not act confident about the decision, the new resident will sense that and feel insecure about the environment.

Once the primary caregiver feels at ease with the transition, often times the loved one will adapt successfully, as well.

4.   What are the most common mistakes a caregiver makes in her attempt to care for a loved one at home?

DONNA FINTO-BURKS, *Nurse Manager:*

The most common mistake is not including the family member who has dementia in conversations and decisions. Examples of this include not offering choices, speaking about the patient as if she is not present. Another misstep is acting frustrated with the loved one as a result of forgetting it's the disease, not the person, causing the undesirable behavior or forgetfulness. It's never helpful to remind the AD patient what he used to be able to do. Many caregivers miss the joy that comes from simply enjoying their loved one where they are at this stage of their life. Caregivers neglecting their own health and need for rest and relaxation is probably the most common mistake.

JUDY GIVEN, *Director of Campus Development:*

People struggle to communicate with their loved one with dementia. A lack of understanding about how that individual is (or isn't) processing your words and actions can exacerbate a challenging situation. Participating in support groups and attending workshops on understanding dementia are often helpful. There, well-trained and experienced caregivers demonstrate useful techniques.

BRENDA NAGEY, *Director of Life Engagement:*
Common mistakes include:

• Not giving a loved one with dementia purpose or making them feel needed. These individuals are still able and interested in doing small tasks, so encourage them to do what they still can. Don't worry about completing the task: enjoying it and feeling purposeful are the goal.

• Rushing a person with dementia. They sense your frustration, and it makes them feel they have disappointed you.

• Arguing. For example, instead of saying "We aren't going to church today, it's Monday!" say, "Maybe later, right now I need your help setting the table."

• Saying "No" or using other negative responses. Instead of saying "You did that wrong," set the object or activity to the side and say, "Thanks for your help." Instead of saying "You can't do that anymore," say, "Today I need your help with folding the towels," or, "I don't need that today. Let's do it tomorrow." You can also try to break the task into smaller, achievable parts and then thank them for their help. This will help them feel purposeful and consequently positive.

• Using too many words. Key words and simple sentences are preferable. For instance, "Honey, dinner," or "Honey, come here please," are preferable to "Honey, you need to come here, wash your hands, and sit down, because it's time to eat. I know you like meatloaf. Come try it." Remember, simple and short.

• Plunking the person with dementia in front of a television for hours on end. Keep them busy, but not simply watching a television. Give them something to hold or touch or do. Activities can include:

Possible Activities:

• Playing dominoes with no rules

• Matching UNO cards

• Matching playing cards

• Playing Black Jack (counting to 21)

• Playing War card game (highest card wins)

• Crocheting a chain

• Clipping coupons

• Signing birthday cards

• Reading aloud

• Singing

• Washing the leaves of fake plants

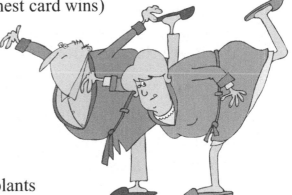

- Polishing shoes or silver or dusting
- Shredding paper

BEVERLY THEIS, *Licensed Social Worker:*
Caregiver burnout is extremely common. Caregivers must take care of their own needs first. Getting respite or enrolling your loved one in a dementia daycare or residential program at least one day a week is a way to take care of yourself. Ask for and be willing to take help when it is offered. Become a part of a caregiving team rather than the sole caregiver. When family caregivers take care of themselves, it frequently improves the relationship with their memory-challenged loved one because they no longer feel resentful and worn-out.

5. What are the most helpful suggestions you can make for those who must care for their loved one at home?

BRENDA NAGEY, *Director of Life Engagement:*
Go to support group meetings and watch the free caregiving videos on Abe's Garden's YouTube channel.

BEVERLY PATNAIK, *Dir. of Staff Training and Community Ed:*
Schedule regular times for meals, bathing, and toileting; choose times when your loved one is most calm. Remove things that may endanger your loved one, such as knives, car keys, guns, and matches. Provide limited choices: For example: two sets of clothes rather than the entire wardrobe, and two choices for a meal. Give instructions one step at a time.

6. What are the most popular activities at Abe's Garden?

BRENDA NAGEY, *Director of Life Engagement:*
The most popular engagement activities at Abe's Garden include drum circle, travel club, singalongs, hand bell choir, current events discussion, Bible study, men's club, themed tea parties, culinary club, flower arranging, setting

tables, folding napkins, caring for the pet dog and cat (brushing and feeding), watching birds in the aviary and hummingbirds at the feeders, art and writing clubs, and spending time outdoors when weather permits.

7. How can a caregiver bring joy to a person with dementia?

BRENDA NAGEY, *Director of Life Engagement:*
Simple things include: sing with them, hold their hand, rub scented lotion on their hands, feed them pudding, brush and style their hair, make them laugh, ask for their opinion and thank them, tell them they are needed and helpful, say "please" and "thank you," call them by the name they prefer, know what they like and have an interest in, read to them, show them YouTube videos of things related to their past, show them pictures of family and talk to them about good times, sit on the porch with them, play familiar music, tell stories from their past, read them the "Dear Abby" advice column and ask what they would do, read sports news to them, have them help you fold a sheet or towels, have them help you stir the pudding for dessert or frost a cake. In short, include them in your daily life.

BEVERLY PATNAIK, *Dir. of Staff Training and Community Ed.:*
Begin each interaction with a smile, then engage their senses, for instance: feel and smell fresh herbs and flower petals, tell the person with dementia what a splendid and good person they are, sit outside and watch and listen to the birds or squirrels. Remember that it's not what you say, but how you make a person feel that lingers. Be encouraging.

8. Any tips on dealing with sun-downing?

DONNA FINTO-BURKS, *Nurse Manager:*
Structure, structure, structure. People with dementia need predictability. Avoid planning family gatherings or social events during the hours your loved one sun-downs, if possible. Help your loved one focus on things they still can do.

9. Any tips for when the patient refuses to bathe or eat?

CHRIS COELHO, *Cont. Ed. and Quality Improvement Coordinator:*

• Try not doing it all at once. Each type of care, or even washing each body part, can be addressed at different times throughout the day, or throughout the week.

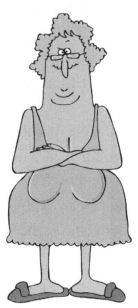

• Take a step back, assess the true cause of the refusal, then adapt the task to the person. For bathing, the issue may be the temperature of the water, the temperature of the room, fear of running water, or modesty about being seen naked. Adjust the temperature of the room and water, try using no-rinse shampoo and soap, and cover her private areas with a towel.

• For eating refusals, consider whether it is certain foods they are refusing, the time the food is being offered, or how difficult the food is to eat. Try offering foods the person enjoys eating, prepare foods so they are easier to chew, adjust the time the meal is served, or serve smaller portions more often throughout the day.

• Adapt every situation to the patient's needs, preference, and capabilities for the stage of Alzheimer's they are in.

10. Any tips on inappropriate comments or violent behavior?

DONNA FINTO-BURKS, *Nurse Manager:*

Don't approach someone from the back or touch them without speaking first, always speak respectfully, and redirect their focus. In addition, evaluate their medications and try identifying potential triggers.

11. After years of caring for people with dementia, tell us some suggestions or advice most caregivers don't know. What have you and your staff learned the hard way?

CHRIS COELHO, *Cont. Ed. and Quality Improvement Coordinator*
Ask yourself why it's important for the patient to do a certain task or why they can't do it. Slow down and don't rush. Educate yourself about the disease and learn from others—you don't have to develop every solution yourself.

DONNA FINTO-BURKS, *Nurse Manager:*
Patience, patience, patience. Use all your senses to relate to your loved one. Listen, look in her eyes, smile, pat her hand, sing her favorite song.

12. **What are your top three suggestions for caregivers?**

DONNA FINTO-BURKS, *Nurse Manager:*

- Be ready to learn.
- Live in the moment.
- Dance and sing a lot.

BEVERLY PATNAIK, *Dir. of Staff Training and Community Ed.:*

- Don't try to reason, argue or correct a person with dementia. You cannot change their reality. You must be the one to change.
- You cannot control the disease—only your response to the disease.
- Every day will be different—what works one day may not work the next. Keep numerous options in your toolkit.

BEVERLY THEIS, *Licensed Social Worker:*

- Every day is a new day. Start afresh each day with a positive attitude.
- Make a memory with your loved one.
- Things can be learned. New hobbies and interests can be found. Try to keep the patient engaged.

13. Any tips on communicating?

BEVERLY PATNAIK, *Dir. of Staff Training and Community Ed:*
Communicating with a person with dementia can be challenging. But there are several things you can do to make communication more successful.

Communication Tips:

- Don't ask if they remember something or someone.

- Introduce yourself every time and call the person by their preferred name.

- Use simple sentences and provide one instruction at a time.

- Ask questions simply, one at a time, and with only two answer options.

- Give the person plenty of time to process the question before expecting a response.

- Offer invitations as opposed to requests.

- Encourage reminiscences even if the memories are not factual.

- Ask permission prior to helping the patient perform a task. Apologize when confronted with anger, insults, or accusations.

- Spark conversation by giving them hints. "The ham we had at Cracker Barrel was wonderful. What do you suppose made it so tasty?" You're not really looking for answers, you're looking to continue a relationship, and conversation is a way to do that. Give maximum information and expect minimum responses.

- Non-verbal communication is important. Make eye contact, keep environmental distractions like TV volume to a minimum, and use hands and touch to guide the patient.

- Pay attention to body language—both yours and the patients. Patients often provide non-verbal cues to reveal they need to use the restroom or feel hungry.

For more tips on communicating with dementia patients, go to You Tube and search for Abe's Garden, Extended: Communicating and Alzheimer's Disease.

14. Any tips on successfully engaging with the patient?

BEVERLY PATNAIK, *Dir. of Staff Training and Community Ed:*

People with dementia depend on their caregivers to make their life meaningful. Engagements are going to be radically different from the beginning stage to the end stage, but it's always going to build on relationship.

While they may be forgetting what they like or don't like, caregivers can remember that for them and use every day things to engage and enhance the relationship. Think about the daily activities they can be a part of in some way. For example, have the person with dementia scoop batter when making cookies. Invite them to participate according to their capabilities.

For more tips on engaging people with dementia, go to You Tube and search for Abe's Garden, Extended: One-on-One Engagement.

What should family members look for in a memory care center or residential community?

JUDY GIVEN, *Director of Campus Development:*

A lot of factors are involved in selecting a memory care community that is right for your family. *How to Evaluate the Quality of Residential Care for Persons with Dementia* is a valuable resource to guide families through this process. It is available as a free, digital download from the Abe's Garden website at: abesgarden.org. Once there, click the "Resources" link, then the "Evaluating Care" link. Printed copies may be requested by contacting Abe's Garden directly.

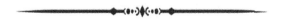

PART IV

HOPE FOR THE FUTURE

CHAPTER 35

RESEARCH—HOPE FOR THE FUTURE
Dr. Sally Burbank

Alzheimer's disease and similar dementias currently have no cure, and despite over 400 clinical trials of promising new Alzheimer's treatments, not a single new drug since 2003 has proven more effective than a placebo. After fifteen years with no cure or new medication, is there any hope for a breakthrough?

Yes, and here's why: According to the Population Reference Bureau, 10,000 baby boomers a day are turning sixty-five. By 2029, there will be over 71 million seniors living in the United States, and this group will comprise a whopping 20% of the population. Skyrocketing rates of dementia, overflowing nursing homes, and a bankrupt Medicaid system will be the result if we don't come up with effective treatments for AD. Already, the U.S spends $200 billion annually on the care of those with dementia, and with the aging baby boomers, this figure will climb to one trillion by 2050. That is roughly equal to our current defense budget!

As a consequence, law makers took note and made Alzheimer's research a top priority in federal medical funding. In 2017, they appropriated 1.4 billion dollars for AD research.

In 2012, the National Alzheimer's Project Act (NAPA) was passed, and their National Plan to Address Alzheimer's Disease was designed to expand and coordinate research. This means a partnership between the government, pharmaceutical companies, non-profit Alzheimer's foundations, and academia was developed to coordinate research and streamline effective early diagnosis and treatment. NAPA's overarching research goal is "to prevent or effectively treat Alzheimer's disease by 2025." For more information you can visit: http://aspe.hhs.gov/national-alzheimers-project-act

---

The Accelerating Medicine Partnership (AMP-AD) is committed to bringing all medications proven to be safe and effective (in double-blinded, placebo-controlled trials) to the FDA for expedited approval.

The United States is not the only country facing skyrocketing rates of Alzheimer's disease. In an effort to coordinate, integrate, and compare research portfolios worldwide, the International Alzheimer's Disease Research Portfolio (IADRP) was developed by the National Institute of Aging. For more information about IADRP visit: http://iadrp.nia.nih.gov

From the research I have reviewed, it is clear that starting medications *after* a patient is already moderately demented is not the answer: it can only delay the progression by about six months. By the time the disease gets diagnosed, too much of the brain has already degenerated. In short—too little, too late. This may be why none of the 400 research trials since 2003 have found an effective treatment. Thus, the greatest advances will have to be in *early* detection and *early* treatment, when there is more viable brain tissue to save.

Let's think about what early detection might look like:

Since 55 to 60% of Alzheimer's patients have inherited at least one copy of the Apolipoprotein E4 allele, (which can be detected cheaply with a simple blood test), what if we started screening for Apo E-4 at age twenty? Since those carrying this allele have an increased risk for AD, (3x the risk with one allele and 10x the risk with two), we could stress risk factor reduction in this group and monitor them carefully, checking blood pressure, LDL cholesterol, exercise habits, smoking habits, and encouraging a strict Mediterranean diet. Careful monitoring and compliance by the individual could lower or delay the risk of developing Alzheimer's. In addition, we could target research trials for early detection and treatment using this group of higher-risk individuals long before any cognitive decline occurs.

Unfortunately, early detection is not as easy as screening everyone for the Apo E4 allele. Forty percent of AD patients do not carry an Apo E-4 allele, and the majority of people with Apo E4 do not get Alzheimer's—they are merely at increased risk. Thus, what we need is a test to determine which individuals are on a likely trajectory to developing Alzheimer's and which are not.

What is being done in the area of early detection?

The greatest goal of research today is to discover which biomarkers or imaging studies can pick up those individuals at high risk for Alzheimer's *before* any brain degeneration has occurred, as this is when intervention will be most effective.

I am encouraged with recent PET scans, (which are still experimental and NOT available at your local radiology center), that are investigating accumulation of beta-amyloid and tau proteins in the brains of patients long before they show clinical signs of disease. Those who develop AD *after* age sixty-five show accumulation of tau protein in the medial temporal lobe and hippocampus, while those who develop AD *before* age sixty-five show tau accumulation in different parts of the brain.

Gerard Bischof, a Ph.D. from the University of Cologne in Germany, is having success using an investigational isotope during PET scans to locate and quantify neurofibrillary tangles in the brain, which are a marker of Alzheimer's disease. In the past, neurofibrillary tangles could only be discovered at autopsy.

Other PET scan isotopes have shown increased tau protein and decreased metabolic activity in the hippocampus and medial temporal lobes in very early-stage Alzheimer's patients—changes which were not seen in the control group. Other PET scan studies are concentrating on how early in the disease process beta-amyloid can be detected in the brain, and how much beta-amyloid is raised simply from age alone rather than dementia.

We now need large, long-term clinical trials to follow those with seemingly normal brains, using these special PET scans, so we can determine when the earliest signs of brain degeneration can be detected. I am happy to report these studies are being done at several research centers throughout the U.S. In fact, I have personally volunteered to be included in a trial through the Alzheimer's

Disease Neuroimaging Initiative (ADNI). If you are interested in participating, visit their website www.adni-info.org and contact them to see if you qualify for the study.

There is a downside to relying on special PET scans, however. The tests are expensive, they last two hours, and the AV-1451 isotope is still investigational and not available to the general public at routine radiology centers. Also, the study I am participating in requires a spinal tap every year. (I'm not looking forward to that!)

To make a definitive biological diagnosis of Alzheimer's, there are currently three cerebrospinal fluid biomarkers: amyloid-B1-42 peptide, T-tau, and P-tau. Levels of these biomarkers can also demonstrate progression from mild cognitive impairment to full-blow AD. Levels of amyloid-B1-42 peptide drops to half normal in AD patients compared to elderly controls, while T-tau and P-tau increase by 200-300%. Unfortunately, most patients will not be willing to get the required spinal tap to be screened in this manner, however.

What is really needed is a simple blood test that will pick up future Alzheimer's patients years before they show evidence of the disease, since that is when interventions would be most effective. There is currently no such test. One of the obstacles to developing such a test is the "blood-brain barrier," which separates the brain from the bloodstream. A patient could have a normal level in the bloodstream, but a low level in the brain. Coming up with an early-detection Alzheimer's test is an ongoing area of research.

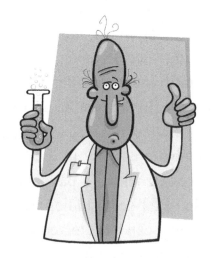

If you would like to participate in reputable research trials about dementia, go to the clinicaltrials.gov website and see if there is a research site near you.

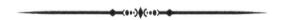

Are there any promising future AD treatments?

The most promising research I have seen is with the use of an antisense oligonucleotide injection. Trials in mice and monkeys have shown a reduction of tau deposits and neuronal loss in the brain. (DeVos, Sl et al., Science Translation Med, 9 (2017)). This infusion may have to be injected into the spinal fluid to be effective, and no human studies have been completed. Time will tell if this is another disappointing wild goose chase.

In November of 2017, Microsoft co-founder, Bill Gates, pledged $100 million to Alzheimer's research through the Dementia Discovery Fund. It turns out that several of Gate's elderly relatives suffered with dementia.

Scientists at the Vanderbilt Center for Neuroscience Drug Discovery have worked on a new molecule, VU319, that looks promising. They are already performing Phase I (early stage) trials in humans.

After the untimely death of beloved University of Tennessee women's basketball coach, Pat Summit, to Alzheimer's, The Pat Summit Clinic was established in Knoxville to provide treatment and research. In short, reputable clinics and research centers are cropping up everywhere, and the National Institute of Aging will try to coordinate and consolidate the research results.

What about stem cell transplantation?

Can stem cells be induced to replace the damaged or dead neurons that are destroyed by AD?

The brains of mammals contain a small number of neural stem cells (NSCs) that can differentiate into any kind of cell in the central nervous system. In a recent research trial, NSC-derived cholinergic neurons and choline acetyltransferase (a neurotransmitter) were able to restore the cognitive performance and synaptic integrity in the brains of rodents with AD. Unfortunately, there are only a few neural stem cells in brain tissue. But, if their proliferation could be induced with growth factors and epigenetic manipulations, this might develop into an effective treatment down the line even for those with moderate or more severe Alzheimer's.

Besides NSCs, there are three other kinds of stem cells—mesenchymal, embryonic, and induced pluripotent. These types are more plentiful than neural stem cells, but they may need careful genetic HLA matching to prevent rejection by the immune system, allergic reactions, or tumor formation. Because of this possibility, human trials are proceeding cautiously.

Speaking of caution... All stem cell research related to brain disorders in humans is in its infancy, and most research is still at the stage of animal trials. Greedy charlatans, however, are duping desperate Alzheimer's patients and their families into spending small fortunes on supposedly miraculous stem cell treatments. These insufficiently tested and non-FDA-approved treatments work no better than placebos at this point. Don't fall for it! Unless it is a legitimate stem cell study being sponsored by the National Institutes of Aging or some reputable medical center, (following scientific standards of using a placebo group for comparison and double-blinding), it is not worth pursuing. You should not have to PAY to be in a research trial. Also, if you are considering some herbal supplement or experimental treatment, discuss it with your neurologist first.

After death, the brains of Alzheimer's patients are often found at autopsy to have other causes for dementia, such as mini strokes, small vessel ischemia (due to high blood pressure or high cholesterol), or previous head trauma. Thus, dementia is not always an "either/or" proposition. As patients age, all of the insults to the brain that have accumulated over a lifetime add up. This explains why in identical twins one may get dementia and the other may not, or one may develop it ten years before the other.

In short, we must do everything we can to protect our brains by keeping our blood pressure and cholesterol in check, eating a Mediterranean diet, exercising regularly, wearing bike helmets if we ride, staying socially active, and stimulating our brains with challenging activities. There is still much for our dedicated researchers to uncover, but in the meantime, we should take brain health seriously.

Lastly, the National Institute of Aging is the leading NIH institute for AD research, and their website is a great resource. I encourage you to follow this site because it provides the most recent and promising research results as they unfold. Here is their website: https://www.nia.nih.gov/health/alzheimers

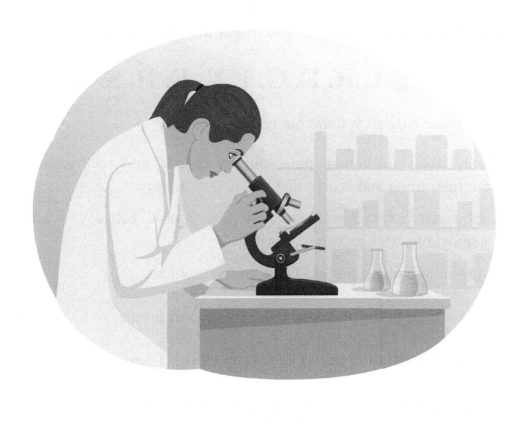

FINAL NOTE FROM THE AUTHORS

We hope a cure for dementia is found soon so the suffering endured by patients and caregivers is eradicated. Until then, we wish you all the best as you navigate the choppy waters of caregiving. We hope at least some of our advice proves helpful. Pick out that which helps, ignore that which doesn't, and be sure to consult with your physician for the final word.

Here is an acronym to remind you of our most salient advice:

~ C. A. R. E. G. I. V. E. R. S. ~

Coordinate care so you are not responsible 24/7.

Accept that you cannot pull your loved one into reality. Instead, put yourself into their mind and accept that this is their reality.

Rest and relax. Schedule an hour a day or a half-day a week to do something enjoyable. Make sleep a priority.

Enjoy simple pleasures and living in the moment.

Groups. Find or develop a caregiver's support group.

Investigate what to expect at each stage of the disease.

Vent. Alzheimer's patients can try your patience, so have a trusted friend to whom you can vent so you won't be short with your loved one.

Exercise. Walk, dance, or join a class at the YMCA. Exercise helps combat depression. A walking buddy is ideal.

Research local adult daycares, respite centers, cleaning services, grocery or pharmacy delivery services. Find trusted back-up.

Schedule your day so you can accomplish all the "have-to" chores as well as an hour a day of "me" time. Get organized and consolidate errands.

ADDITIONAL RESOURCES

Alzheimer's Association: This non-profit not only raises money for Alzheimer's research, but also provides resources. Contact them to locate a support group near you or to get help starting a group in your community.

Alzheimer's Association
225 N Michigan Ave, Floor 17
Chicago, IL 60601-5997

Telephone: (800) 272-3900
Website: www.alz.org.

EXCELLENT BOOKS

- *The 36-Hour Day* by Nancy Mace and Peter Rabins

- *The Dementia Caregiver* by Marc Agronin

- *Alzheimer's Disease: Unraveling the Mystery* by National Institutes of Health, 2008. Download this free publication in a PDF format or order a print copy from the National Institute on Aging website.

- *Learning to Speak Alzheimer's* by Robert N. Butler, M.D

- *A Pocket Guide for the Alzheimer's Caregiver* by Daniel C. Potts MD and Ellen Woodward Potts

PART V

STORIES FROM
Patient's I Will Never Forget

◆⟨••⟩◗◖⟨••⟩◆

The following three stories are taken from Dr. Burbank's book, *Patients I Will Never Forget*, which is available through Amazon.com in paperback and Kindle form. These three stories all involve caretaking patients with Alzheimer's disease.

HOW I OUTSMARTED
A PACK OF RAVENOUS WOLVES

A true story by Dr. Sally Willard Burbank

Edgar Summers, a patient with severe Alzheimer's disease, was convinced wolves were prowling outside the hospital waiting for him to fall asleep so they could sneak in and gobble him up. Nurse Ratchet had already tried reasoning with him, but Edgar became more agitated and accused her of wanting him eaten so she could admit another patient and make more money.

A nurse's aide tried to calm Edgar down by telling him she had sent a security officer outside to take care of the wolves. Big mistake! Edgar was now convinced the security officer had been eaten alive. Nurse Ratchet paged the security officer to Edgar's room to reassure him he was unharmed and had scared away the wolves.

Edgar insisted the wolves would soon be back. At this point, Nurse Ratchet paged me and wanted me to prescribe a shot of Haldol, a potent anti-psychotic, to simmer down his paranoia and put him to sleep.

Before resorting to medications, which can increase the risk of falls and hip fractures in the elderly, I wanted to try one more non-pharmaceutical approach.

I knew telling Edgar there were no wolves was pointless because, in his mind, the wolves were real. Thus, arguing with him would prove as productive as Congressional budget negotiations. While some may consider it lying, I knew the way to calm Edgar was to put myself in his mind and then try to outsmart the wolves.

With this understanding of severe Alzheimer's disease, I pulled up a chair next to Edgar's bed and told him I knew of a foolproof method to protect him and all the other patients in the hospital from the vicious wolves outside.

I shared with Edgar that every hospital door had a four-digit security code; the doors wouldn't open unless the secret code was entered.

"Edgar," I whispered conspiratorially, "I'm going to change the security

---

code. If the wolves don't know the code, the doors won't open, and they can't get in."

His brow furrowed as he tried to understand. "You'll use a code the wolves don't know, and I'll be safe?"

"Exactly, and I'll even let you pick the four numbers. That way, only you and I know the numbers."

He smiled, and his face visibly relaxed. He whispered four arbitrary numbers into my ear, and I left to go supposedly change the security code. When I came back fifteen minutes later to check on him, he was sound asleep.

My clever scheme had worked … until the next night when Edgar insisted an angry clan of rhinos would charge into the hospital using their horns to smash down the doors! Thus, changing the security code wouldn't protect him. But that's fodder for another story!

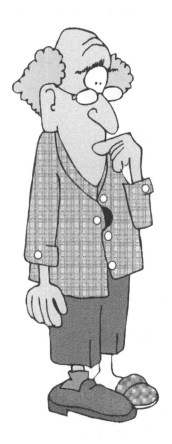

"His memory is like wares at an auction— going, going, gone."

~ Herman Melville~

THE SPIDER ON THE WALL

A true story by Dr. Sally Willard Burbank

At age ninety, Cora Jones suffered moments when her memory failed. She'd lose her nephew's name, the gist of Sunday's sermon, what she ate for lunch, and what her daughter told her she wanted for Christmas. Thus, when she was admitted to the hospital for emergency gall bladder surgery, no one was surprised when she couldn't remember the name of her blood pressure pill or the name of her surgeon. The admitting nurse quickly concluded Cora must have early Alzheimer's, and she passed along her suspicion to Nurse Ratchet, who'd been scheduled for the night shift.

Thus, when Cora pushed the nurse button to report a huge spider crawling on the ceiling above her head, Nurse Ratchet didn't take her seriously. "The woman is obviously sun downing," she informed the unit clerk, then cranked down Cora's morphine drip. That'll take care of the spider.

Thirty minutes later, Cora rattled her bed rails and mashed on the nurse button again. "I can't sleep with the big spider glaring down at me. It could be a brown recluse waiting to bite me," she insisted.

Hmm. She didn't have any trouble remembering the words "brown recluse."

But Nurse Ratchet was convinced the morphine was making Cora see things, and now she was even paranoid. She came into the room and turned off the morphine drip and patted Cora's hand. "There, there, dearie. There's no spider; it's just your morphine drip making you hallucinate."

She informed Cora she'd call the surgeon to order something to take care of her hallucinations.

"I don't need drugs!" Cora fumed. "I need you to kill that spider!"

Cora refused to take the anti-psychotic medication. Nurse Ratchet patted her hands in a patronizing manner and quickly exited the room, refusing to validate Cora's imaginary spider by actually inspecting the ceiling.

When I entered Cora's room on rounds the next morning, the first words out of her mouth were, "I couldn't sleep a wink with that huge spider over my bed." She crossed her arms in disgust. "That nurse didn't believe a word I said. Instead, she turned off my pain medication, and now I hurt so bad I can hardly get out of bed. She should be fired!"

I glanced up at the ceiling to inspect for a spider just to prove Cora wrong. I nearly dropped my morning coffee when, on the ceiling directly above Cora's head, I spied a large brown spider, sitting in the middle of his web! Cora pointed at the arachnid accusingly. "I told that nurse there was a spider! She wouldn't even look!"

Not a spider fan myself, I called housekeeping to come remove the NOT-SO-IMAGINARY spider!

Revenge is sweet…and not fattening!

Alfred Hitchcock

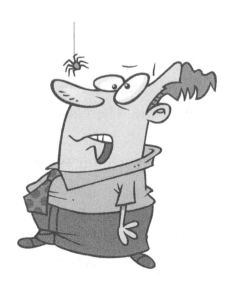

BAD, BAD LEROY BROWN

A true story by Dr. Sally Willard Burbank

Worry lines creased Marsha's forehead. "I swear, my father won't die of Alzheimer's—I'm going to kill him first!"

Sensing she needed to vent about the challenges of caring for her demented father, I invited Marsha to clue me in.

At ninety-four, Leroy Brown—name changed to protect the guilty—had trash and junk piled to the ceiling of his Detroit home. The only food in the refrigerator was beer and moldy pizza. He hadn't taken his blood pressure pill in months, and the electric department had turned off his power for nonpayment. He'd recently gotten confused driving home from the grocery store and ended up two counties away and out of gas. In short, his Alzheimer's disease had progressed to the point where he could no longer care for himself.

Marsha flew to Detroit and located a competent nurse's aide to cook, clean, pay bills, and keep an eye on him.

Two days later, however, the aide called to resign. Why? Every time she attempted to show up for work, Leroy brandished a rifle at her and hollered, "Get your fat a** off my property, or I'll shoot!"

Marsha flew back to Detroit, confiscated the rifle, and came up with Plan B. This time, she dug up a caregiver who agreed to move into the house in exchange for free rent and food. Marsha helped her settle into the guest bedroom. "Don't you worry," she insisted, patting Marsha's hand. "I've dealt with plenty of Alzheimer's patients before. I'm sure I can handle him."

Three weeks later, however, the caregiver called and was moving out—today! The old geezer had exposed himself on multiple occasions and now was groping her and insisting if she was going to live in his house, she had better earn her keep—and he didn't mean by cleaning the toilet.

Marsha flew back to Detroit for a third time. She moved him into an assisted-living program against his will.

A week later, she received a frantic call from the facility. "Leroy crawled out of his second story window using his sheet as a rope. We have no idea where he is."

Since it was nighttime in the dead of winter, the police were called to help locate him before he froze to death. Eight hours later, they found him all right—warm and toasty—watching television in his recliner back at his old house.

Even though the assisted-living facility was four miles away, he had apparently walked in his bathrobe and slippers until "some guy in a truck" offered him a ride. Leroy made no apology for the angst he'd caused. "It's your own &%$# fault," he hissed at his daughter. "I told you I didn't want to live in that old folks' home."

Fed up with his tomfoolery, Marsha admitted him to a nursing home that locked its front door and had no windows from which he could crawl out. Before the day was over, nurses scolded him for profane language, pinching and groping the nurses, and flinging Brussels sprouts at a chatty patient in the dining room who grated on his nerves. Another day, he stuffed a sock in the mouth of a fellow Alzheimer's patient. "It's her own *&%# fault," he snapped at the nurse. "I told her to shut up, but she wouldn't stop hollering."

Then the unthinkable happened. Late one night, another nursing home resident, Mr. Williams, became confused and shuffled with his walker into Leroy's room by mistake.

Startled by the "prowler," Leroy picked up his cane and began clobbering the poor man. The nurse on duty heard the commotion and ran into the room just in time to witness Mr. Williams thrusting his walker—its legs directed toward Leroy—as though it were a shield. Leroy struck back with his cane, as though it were a sword.

Before the nurse could stop him, Leroy administered such a hard whack that both men landed on the floor in a heap. Security broke up the brawl, and Mr. Williams was ambulanced to the hospital for X-rays. Leroy managed to escape unscathed, but he refused to apologize. Arms crossed, he insisted, "It was his fault. He shouldn't have been prowling around my room. I thought he was a burglar."

———

Right! A ninety-five-year-old burglar with a walker?

After Leroy's latest antics, thoughts of patricide entered Marsha's head. What was she going to do with the incorrigible old cuss?

Because of the brawl, Leroy was kicked out of the nursing home and admitted to the psychiatric ward for evaluation. As though sensing he was doomed for powerful psych drugs or electric shock treatment if he didn't behave himself, Leroy suddenly became a model patient: pleasant, clean-mouthed, and he even managed to keep his hands to himself. When Marsha walked in, he had the nurses and doctors on the psych ward in stitches with his humorous tales from World War II.

He had hoodwinked them all. The psychiatrist remarked, "Leroy was just defending himself from a man he thought was a prowler." The doctor then went on to insist, "He's acting out because he needs more activity and stimulation."

Leroy heartily agreed, as he ogled the attractive nurse standing nearby. He then turned to Marsha and scolded, "I told you nothing was wrong with me. You're the one with the problem."

The problem was hers all right—what to do with Leroy! If he didn't straighten up soon, she would land in the psych ward with a mental breakdown. Or jail—for murder!

The first nursing home refused to take Leroy back. After begging and pleading, Marsha cajoled another nursing home into admitting Leroy. At the advice of the psychiatrist, he was enrolled in stimulating activities, such as arts and crafts, shuffleboard, and physical therapy.

Unfortunately, he was banned from arts and crafts after offending the lady participants with his vulgar crayon drawing of a voluptuous nude woman. He was banned from shuffleboard after he lost a game, flung his cue in a fit of rage, and broke it. His stick had missed another resident's head by mere inches.

Maybe physical therapy would be the ticket …

The physical therapist enrolled Leroy in a program using elastic bands and five-pound weights. Since Leroy also suffered from arthritis in his knees, the therapist focused on strengthening his quadriceps.

One day, Leroy wasn't in the mood for therapy and refused to participate.

"Come on, Leroy, it'll be good for you," the therapist encouraged.

"I don't want to." He pursed his lips and crossed his arms like a petulant child.

"You can do it," the therapist encouraged. "I insist you at least give it a try." He pulled Leroy off the bed and into a standing position. "Therapy will strengthen your knees."

Annoyed that the therapist hadn't listened to him, Leroy walloped his bent knee straight into the crotch of the therapist.

The poor therapist howled and doubled over in pain, as Leroy snapped, "Nothing wrong with that knee. Want me to show you how well the other knee works, too?"

The therapist limped from the room and refused to EVER work with Leroy again. Marsha was, yet again, called—like she knew how to control her father!

"What can I do?" she snapped at the head of the nursing home. "I'm here in Nashville, and I can't afford to miss any more work. He is costing me a fortune in plane tickets. Deal with it." She slammed down the phone, frustrated beyond measure.

Leroy was sent back to the psych ward, but this time they prescribed potent medications to keep him calm. While she hated the thought of him all doped up, at least no more people ended up in the ER—or sterilized. Once sedated, he was sent back to the nursing home, this time compliant.

"My short-term memory is bad...
And so is my short-term memory."
~Bill Murray~

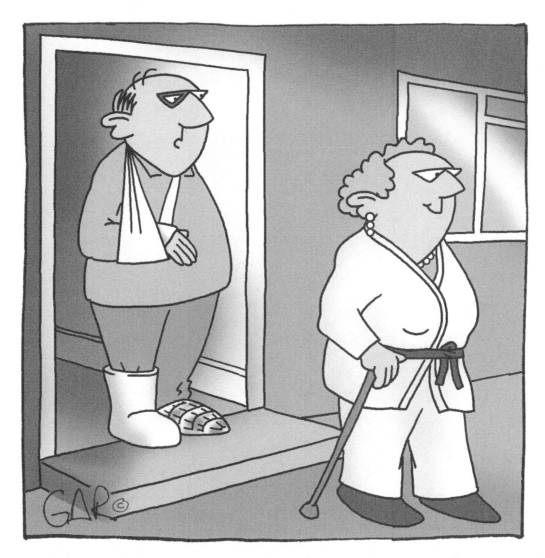

"Darling, I wish you'd stop the self defense classes, now you've got Alzheimer's."

Made in the USA
Coppell, TX
01 July 2021